Handbook of
HEADACHE MANAGEMENT

A Practical Guide to Diagnosis and
Treatment of Head, Neck, and Facial Pain

Handbook of
HEADACHE MANAGEMENT

A Practical Guide to Diagnosis and Treatment of Head, Neck, and Facial Pain

Joel R. Saper, M.D.,

Stephen D. Silberstein, M.D.

C. David Gordon, M.D.

Robert L. Hamel, P.A.-C

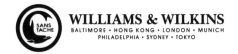

WILLIAMS & WILKINS
BALTIMORE · HONG KONG · LONDON · MUNICH
PHILADELPHIA · SYDNEY · TOKYO

Editor: Jonathan W. Pine, Jr.
Managing Editor: Carol Eckhart
Copy Editor: Judith F. Minkove
Designer: Wilma E. Rosenberger
Illustration Planner: Lorraine Wrzosek
Production Coordinator: Kimberly Nawrozki

Copyright © 1993
Williams & Wilkins
428 East Preston Street
Baltimore, Maryland 21202, USA

Accurate indications, adverse reactions, and dosage schedules for drugs are provided in this book, but it is possible that they may change. The reader is urged to review the package information data of the manufacturers of the medications mentioned.

Printed in the United States of America

Library of Congress Cataloging-in-Publication Data

Handbook of headache management : a practical guide to diagnosis and treatment of head, neck, and facial pain/Joel R. Saper . . . [et al.]
   p.   cm.
   Includes bibliographical references and index.
   ISBN 0-683-05801-0
   1. Headache—Handbooks, manuals, etc. I. Saper, Joel R.
   [DNLM: 1. Facial Pain—diagnosis—handbooks. 2. Facial Pain—therapy—handbooks. 3. Headache—diagnosis—handbooks. 4. Headache—therapy—handbooks. WL 39 H236]
RB128.H35 1993
616.8′491—dc20
DNLM/DLC
for Library of Congress   92-23747
                                                CIP

92 93 94 95 96
1 2 3 4 5 6 7 8 9 10

Preface

This book represents a commitment to physicians and other health care professionals who treat headache disorders and require a practical, efficient manual, addressing the key features of diagnosis and management.

During the past decade, a noteworthy advance in headache treatment has occurred. Though still not a "mainstream" specialty, a growing number of well-trained, dedicated, and scholarly professionals are pursuing the field of headache management. This interest parallels the recognition that pain therapy has been a sadly ignored aspect of medical care. Indeed, the symptoms of pain have not been approached with the same scholarly vigor and intensity that has been accorded far less pervasive and disabling conditions. Shrouded in myth, mistreatment, or neglect, the headache disorders and patients who suffer from them have been confronted in a suboptimal manner.

To arrive at the most practical perspective for this book, many serious challenges arise. There is no widely accepted standard of care for the treatment of persistent or recurring, benign headache. Alas, no particular discipline in medicine has emerged and been acknowledged as the authoritative body for the treatment of this illness. Headache is an "orphan illness," with authorities from a variety of different perspectives and disciplines submitting what they believe to be the pathogenic origin and proper treatment, often in stark contradiction to that of other disciplines.

Thus, the patient with persisting headache is likely to encounter an assembly line of medical care and services and an array of explanations and treatments, many of which are narrowly focused along the lines of subspecialty care and training. From sinus disease to allergy, from mental duress to neck problems, from yeast purging to colon purging, the headache patient has traveled along a pathway of costly and sometimes damaging explanations and services that often aggravate the problem, delay the diagnosis, complicate the eventual treatment, and frustrate everyone.

This book approaches the problem of headache from a neurobiological perspective. The book is not designed as an encyclopedic reference for all aspects of head and neck pain. It assumes some understanding of the problem and emphasizes diagnosis and treatment, providing key information in an easily accessible manner.

We intend to update this manual regularly, remaining vigilant to those trends and acceptable treatments that will aid our colleagues. The reader will note that major portions of this book are presented in outline form, with an abundance of tables. It is hoped that this will facilitate convenience by making material easily accessible and usable.

Throughout this text, the reader will encounter the word "selected" before various listings. The use of this word designates that an arbitrary selection of items has been made. The lists are not necessarily exhaustive and should be used only as a reference and a guide. The reader should use this book for direction only, obtaining additional information from various other authoritative sources and references to supplement the information presented here.

Finally, on a philosophical note, recurring head pain, as we now know it, is most often a chronic illness. The wise clinician must avoid the cynicism and bias that has historically influenced illnesses that are not fully understood at the time treatment is demanded. The integrity of complaints must be trusted, unless compelling support forces an alternate attitude.

Patients suffering from headache and related painful disorders are often desperate and complex, frequently rejected by the health care system and often injured and compromised by a long list of failed and inappropriate treatments. A true test of clinical skill and vigor is the effective management of the needs and agony of these individuals. Taking the patient's symptoms to heart is at the heart of prudent medical care. Ultimately, even those persons with illnesses and symptoms that are not fully understood can be treated effectively and compassionately.

Joel R. Saper, M.D.
Stephen Silberstein, M.D.
C. David Gordon, M.D.
Robert L. Hamel, P.A.-C

Acknowledgments

The authors wish to acknowledge the following individuals:

Debbie Johnston, for her diligent and skillful technical assistance and remarkable endurance, and most of all for her sustaining commitment, friendliness, and charm;

Alvin E. Lake III, Ph.D., with special thanks for the trust and friendship from the very beginning, and particularly for the knowledge, wisdom, and perspective that is so capably shared with colleagues, and without which the Institute and its work could never have been the same;

Grace Lobel, for support and understanding beyond simple description, and for more than 12 years of friendship, devotion, and extraordinary patience;

Marjorie Winters, R.N., B.S.N., for her skillful and diligent help with this manuscript, and for over a decade of prudent advice, dedication, and professional dignity; and finally,

Our many other colleagues, friends, and our families for what they must endure to allow such an effort to happen.

Joel R. Saper, M.D., 1992

About the Authors

Joel R. Saper, M.D., F.A.C.P. is the founder and Director of the Michigan Head·Pain & Neurological Institute in Ann Arbor, Michigan (1978) and its Head·Pain Treatment Unit at Chelsea Community Hospital (1979), the nation's first comprehensive, accredited headache treatment program. A Clinical Professor of Medicine (Neurology) at Michigan State University, Dr. Saper is the past President of the American Association for the Study of Headache and a course director and member of the Education Subcommittee of the American Academy of Neurology. He is a member of the Board and educator in the American Academy of Pain Medicine, and in numerous other medical organizations. Dr. Saper is the editor and primary author of "Topics in Pain Medicine," a monthly professional newsletter, and has authored or coauthored six medical books, in addition to numerous chapters and medical articles. Dr. Saper is an invited speaker and has presented his work internationally to medical and other professional forums. He is a graduate of the University of Illinois School of Medicine and trained in neurology at the University of Michigan, and received his board certification in neurology in 1975.

Stephen D. Silberstein, M.D., F.A.C.P. is the Director of the Comprehensive Headache Center at The Germantown Hospital and Medical Center, Philadelphia, Pennsylvania. He received his M.D. degree from the University of Pennsylvania, where he also completed his medicine and neurology training. Dr. Silberstein received his board certification in neurology in 1975. He completed a Special Fellowship in Neurology at the National Hospital for Nervous Diseases at Queen Square, London, and was a research associate in the Toxicology Laboratory of Clinical Science at the National Institute of Mental Health in Bethesda, Maryland. Dr. Silberstein is Clinical Professor of Neurology at Temple University School of Medicine and is a member of the Board and Scientific Program Chairman of the American Association for the Study of Headache. Dr. Silberstein is coeditor of the 6th edition of Wolff's *Headache*. He has presented his scientific work throughout the world and is a frequent invited lecturer at medical and professional gatherings and educational forums.

C. David Gordon, M.D. is a member of the medical faculty of the Michigan Head·Pain & Neurological Institute and is an attending physician to the Head·Pain Treatment Unit at Chelsea Community Hospital. Dr. Gordon is a graduate of Boston University School of Medicine and completed his residency training in internal medicine at Faulkner Hospital in Boston, Massachusetts. He spent two years in specialty practice at the John R. Graham Headache Centre in Boston, where he also completed a fellowship in headache management. Dr. Gordon has particular interest and experience in the computer application of headache education and clinical care and serves as a primary educational resource at the Institute on the integration of the principles of internal medicine to the treatment and evaluation of headache disorders.

Robert L. Hamel, P.A.-C is currently a clinical associate at the Michigan Head · Pain & Neurological Institute in Ann Arbor and clinical liaison and member of the Management Team at the Head · Pain Treatment Unit at Chelsea Community Hospital. He has extensive experience in the evaluation, treatment, and clinical co-ordination of head-injured patients and is the Clinical Coordinator of the Head Injury Program at the Institute. Mr. Hamel received his Bachelor of Science Degree and Physician's Assistant degree from Mercy College in Detroit, Michigan and has a Bachelor of Arts degree in Psychology and a Masters degree in Management. Mr. Hamel's work has achieved national recognition, and he is frequently an invited guest lecturer on state and national levels, presenting educational seminars and lectures on headache and head injury topics.

Contents

To Our Clinical Colleagues

At the heart of responsible and qualified medical care is the clinician who, armed with wisdom, compassion, and experience, applies the art of medicine to the care of patients. Though it is the scientist who must define objectively the biological markers of disease, it is the clinician who is called upon to give relief and guidance, even in the absence of a charted course.

Indeed, the distinction between objective and subjective disease may not be defined so much by the validity of the symptoms, but by the scientific sophistication during the era in which the disorder occurs. And when circumstances demand a thoughtful response in the absence of objective definition, it is the clinician who must rally to vigorously enlist the most creative of resources to bring comfort and direction to those who seek help.

And what makes so difficult the task of the clinician who endeavors to manage pain is the need to master the diagnosis of hundreds of conditions which can produce it, and then to treat this disruptive disorder in the absence of a full understanding of the process, sufficient tools to overcome it, and minimal knowledge of the complexities of human suffering.

JRS, 1992

1

Epidemiology and Classification of Headache

I. Epidemiology

Seventy-six percent (76%) of women and 57% of men report at least one significant headache per month, and over 90% have experienced a headache in their lifetime (Linet, 1989). Headache prevalence in children increases from 39% at age 6 to 70% by age 15. Moreover, it is estimated that 1 million days of missed school and over 150 million days of lost work per year are attributable to headache. Lost productivity estimates for the United States work force per year range from $6.5 to $17.2 billion.

Among migraine sufferers, 86% of females and 82% of males report some disability with each attack. Thirty-one percent (31%) of persons with headache have regular, periodic functional impairment. Despite the painful and disabling impact of headache, many such patients do not seek medical care. Sixty percent (60%) of females and 70% of males with typical migraine have never been diagnosed properly.

In a recent report from the Centers for Disease Control (1990), a 60% increase in the prevalence of migraine during the years 1980–1989 was noted. Eight percent (8%) of sufferers are hospitalized at least once yearly, and 4% of men and 3% of women have a persistently impaired existence.

Independent of quality of life considerations, it is estimated that the annual cost of a migraine sufferer to employer is from $5256 to $6864 per men and $3168 to $3600 per women.

II. Classification

The *primary headaches*, i.e., migraine and cluster headaches, are those in which no consistently identified organic cause can be determined. *Secondary headaches* are those associated with a variety of organic etiologies.

Until recently, the primary classification of headache was based upon the Ad Hoc Committee Report, published in 1962. Following an international effort engineered by Professor Jes Olesen of Copenhagen, the International Headache Society (IHS) has proposed a new classification on headache, informally known as the International Classification. This comprehensive document attempts to reconcile the many and complex aspects of headache into a usable system. Its ultimate acceptance and usability remain to be defined, but it has, if nothing else, organized headache comprehensively for the first time (see Table 1.1).

The new classification of headache gives more precision to the diagnosis of headache in general, and migraine specifically. Common migraine is now called *migraine without aura* and is defined in terms of duration, quality, and associated findings accompanying each attack.

Classic migraine is now called *migraine with aura*, and the features of the aura are delineated in greater detail.

Tension-type headache is the new term for what has previously been called tension headache, muscle contraction headache, stress headache, and ordinary headache. The classification distinguishes between patients with episodic (acute) tension-type headaches and chronic tension-type headaches, with subclassifications based upon the presence or absence of increased tenderness of the pericranial muscles or increased electromyographic (EMG) activity.

Cluster headache and chronic paroxysmal hemicrania are also classified, as are a variety of miscellaneous conditions and headache phenomena. Thirteen categories of headache are subdivided into 129 different subtypes.

TABLE 1.1.   **NEW INTERNATIONAL HEADACHE SOCIETY CLASSIFICATION OF HEADACHE**

1. Migraine	**3. Cluster headache and chronic**
1.1 Migraine without aura	**paroxysmal hemicrania**
1.2 Migraine with aura	3.1 Cluster headache
1.3 Ophthalmoplegic migraine	3.2 Chronic paroxysmal hemicrania
1.4 Retinal migraine	3.3 Cluster headache-like disorder not
1.5 Childhood periodic syndromes that	fulfilling above criteria
may not be precursors to or	**4. Miscellaneous headaches**
associated with migraine	**unassociated with structural**
1.6 Complications of migraine	**lesion**
1.7 Migrainous disorder not fulfilling	4.1 Idiopathic stabbing headache
above criteria	4.2 External compression headache
2. Tension-type headache	4.3 Cold stimulus headache
2.1 Episodic tension-type headache	4.4 Benign cough headache
2.2 Chronic tension-type headache	4.5 Benign exertional headache
2.3 Headache of the tension-type not	4.6 Headache associated with sexual
fulfilling above criteria	activity

TABLE 1.1. **CONTINUED**

5. Headache associated with head trauma
5.1 Acute post-traumatic headache
5.2 Chronic post-traumatic headache
6. Headache associated with vascular disorders
6.1 Acute ischemic cerebrovascular disease
6.2 Intracranial hematoma
6.3 Subarachnoid hemorrhage
6.4 Unruptured vascular malformation
6.5 Arteritis
6.6 Carotid or vertebral artery pain
6.7 Venous thrombosis
6.8 Arterial hypertension
6.9 Headache associated with other vascular disorder
7. Headache associated with nonvascular intracranial disorder
7.1 High cerebrospinal fluid pressure
7.2 Low cerebrospinal fluid pressure
7.3 Intracranial infection
7.4 Intracranial sarcoidosis and other noninfectious inflammatory diseases
7.5 Headache related to intrathecal injections
7.6 Intracranial neoplasm
7.7 Headache associated with other intracranial disorder
8. Headache associated with substances or their withdrawal
8.1 Headache induced by acute substance use or exposure
8.2 Headache induced by chronic substance use or exposure
8.3 Headache from substance withdrawal (acute use)
8.4 Headache from substance withdrawal (chronic use)
8.5 Headache associated with substances but with uncertain mechanism

9. Headache associated with noncephalic infection
9.1 Viral infection
9.2 Bacterial infection
9.3 Headache related to other infection
10. Headache associated with metabolic disorder
10.1 Hypoxia
10.2 Hypercapnia
10.3 Mixed hypoxia and hypercapnia
10.4 Hypoglycemia
10.5 Dialysis
10.6 Headache related to other metabolic abnormality
11. Headache or facial pain associated with disorder of cranium, neck, eyes, ears, nose, sinuses, teeth, mouth, or other facial or cranial structures
11.1 Cranial bone
11.2 Neck
11.3 Eyes
11.4 Ears
11.5 Nose and sinuses
11.6 Teeth, jaws, and related structures
11.7 Temporomandibular joint disease
12. Cranial neuralgias, nerve trunk pain, and deafferentation pain
12.1 Persistent (in contrast to tic-like) pain of cranial nerve origin
12.2 Trigeminal neuralgia
12.3 Glossopharyngeal neuralgia
12.4 Nervus intermedius neuralgia
12.5 Superior laryngeal neuralgia
12.6 Occipital neuralgia
12.7 Central causes of head and facial pain other than tic douloureux
12.8 Facial pain not fulfilling criteria in groups 11 or 12
13. Headache not classifiable

2

Diagnostic Evaluation of the Patient with Headache

"Patients have illnesses and symptoms long before doctors understand them or have the means to diagnose or treat them."
—Saper, 1992

I. The History

A detailed, comprehensive history is undeniably the most important aspect of establishing the diagnosis of a headache condition.

A. Important Variables

Patients must be specifically asked how many headache patterns (different types of headaches) they experience. The following features must be delineated for each type, where appropriate.

- Date, circumstances, and suddenness of onset;
- Intensity/character of pain;
- Duration of individual attack(s);
- Location(s);
- Frequency of attacks;
- Preceding and accompanying neurological or other physical symptoms;
- Seasonal variations;
- Evolution (progression) in symptoms and/or frequency;
- Provoking/aggravating factors;
- Relief measures;
- Current and past treatments, failed and effective;
- Family history;
- Sleep patterns;
- Occupation;
- Emotional profile; and
- Impairment impact.

The distinction between benign (primary) headaches and those of more serious origin can sometimes be made by a determination of the abruptness of onset (particularly the first headache), more than the severity of pain. Severe headache, escalating in intensity over a minute or two, is of significant concern (see Table 2.1).

TABLE 2.1 **KEY FACTORS DISTINGUISHING PHYSIOLOGICAL (PRIMARY) FROM SECONDARY (ORGANIC) HEADACHE**

1. Abruptness of onset
2. Progression of headache pattern
3. Presence of abnormal neurological or other physical findings
4. Nature of provoking and alleviating factors

TABLE 2.2 **SOME SUSPECTED PROVOKING FACTORS[a] OF HEADACHE (PARTICULARLY MIGRAINE)[b]**

Hormonal changes	Certain foods/ingredients (see Table 2.3)
Oral contraceptives	
Menstruation	Missed meals
Hormonal replacement	Stress, exhilaration, or "letdown"
Amenorrhea	Fluorescent lights
Some medicines	Smoke
Position/exertion	
Weather changes	
Lack of or excessive sleep (i.e., more than customary, such as on weekends)	

[a]See also Table 7.6, Chapter 11
[b]The reliability of any of these factors to provoke a headache remains arguable. Overemphasis of their importance can result in patients feeling guilt for continuing attacks, the origin of which may have little to do with factors under their control. Hormonal factors, excessive sleep, missed meals, alcohol, and weather changes represent the most reliable provoking factors.

B. Provoking Factors ("Triggers")

Primary headaches, such as migraine, can frequently be provoked by characteristic factors, such as menstruation, alcohol, or missing meals. The identification of these factors can help to establish the diagnosis.

Many patients suffer from more than one pattern of pain, and each requires separate delineation. Failure to do so results in an inability to distinguish coexisting entities.

Although most patients with recurring headache experience the affliction because of genetic or acquired biological predisposition, various external and internal events can provoke an individual or series of attacks.

Table 2.2 is a listing of the most commonly cited headache-provoking factors. Table 2.3 lists foods that are frequently identified as provoking headaches.

With respect to caffeine, while modest and moderate caffeine intake (up to 300–400 mg/day) may have no adverse effect on headache patients and may help some, excessive caffeine intake can aggravate and induce headaches. Toxicity

TABLE 2.3. **COMMON FOODS THAT MAY PROVOKE HEADACHE**

Food Type	Examples
Aged cheeses	Cheddar, brick, mozzarella, Gruyère, Stilton, Brie, Camembert, Boursault
Alcohol	Beer, wine (especially red), liquor
Caffeine	Coffee, tea, cola, certain over-the-counter analgesics and other medications (see Table 5.2, Chapter 5 for caffeine content of selected foods and analgesics)
Chocolate	Sweets, foods, drinks
Concentrated sugar	Sweets, cookies, cake
Dairy products	Milk, ice cream, yogurt, cream, cheeses (aged)
Fermented, pickled foods	Herring, sour cream, yogurt, vinegar, marinated meats (cold cuts)
Fruits	Bananas, plantain, avocado, figs, passion fruit, raisins, pineapple, oranges, and most citrus
Meats with nitrites	Bologna, hot dogs, pepperoni, salami, pastrami, bacon, sausages, canned ham, corned beef, smoked fish
Monosodium glutamate (MSG)	Chinese food, Accent, Lawry's Seasoned Salt, instant foods such as canned soup, TV dinners, processed meats, roasted nuts, potato chips
Nutrasweet/saccharin	Soft drinks, diet foods
Sulfites	Salad bars, shrimp, soft drinks, certain wines
Vegetables	Onions, pods of broad beans (lima, navy), pea pods, nuts, peanuts
Yeast products	Yeast extract, fresh breads, raised coffee cakes, doughnuts

from caffeine can produce a headache as one of its symptoms. Moreover, high daily chronic intake greater than 500 mg/day can produce dependency, leading to "withdrawal" headaches 8–16 hours after the last dose. This is a major cause of morning headaches in people with large caffeine intake. Table 5.2 in Chapter 5 lists the caffeine content of various foods and drugs. The total daily caffeine intake should be calculated or at least carefully estimated, since caffeine overuse can be important contributing factor in some cases.

II. The Physical Examination

The physical examination, particularly of the head and neck, is an essential element in a comprehensive evaluation for headache. It may be critical in the identification of alternate conditions that may mimic or coexist with a primary headache syndrome and that would otherwise not be identified were careful evaluation not carried out.

In patients with primary headache disorders, except for the occasional presence of "soft neurological signs," the neurological and general examinations are usually normal, as is the neurodiagnostic evaluation. Exceptions occur. For example, neurological findings are sometimes present during *migraine with aura*, and drooping eyelid (ptosis) and pupillary changes are frequently seen during cluster headache. Occipitocervical tenderness is common in migraine and its variants, and the EEG may be mildly abnormal in up to 30–40% of patients with migraine.

The details of a physical/neurological examination will not be listed in this manual. Neurological function and assessment of carotid and temporal artery pulsations, cardiac and peripheral vascular status, and spinal anatomy and function must be carefully determined.

Special attention must be paid to the following aspects of the clinical examination:

- Palpation/percussion
    cranium
    jaw
    neck
    oral cavity
    ears
    sinuses;
- Vital signs
- Mental status
- Funduscopic exam
- Visual acuity
- Signs of trauma
- Cardiac and pulmonary status.

Pathological processes in and about the head or neck can provoke secondary headaches and also activate primary headaches, such as migraine. *Thus, even in the presence of obvious migraine, a careful search for accompanying or inciting illness is necessary.*

Nuchal rigidity can be an important sign of infectious, structural, or hemorrhagic events, but may not be initially evident. *It may take as many as six hours for subarachnoid blood, e.g., from an aneurysm, to migrate to the cervical region and induce the irritational changes that provoke nuchal rigidity (which must be distinguished from muscle tenderness and guarding).* Thus, the absence of neck stiffness does not exclude one of these processes.

III. Laboratory Testing

Over 300 causes of secondary headache are known. (See Table 4.1, Chapter 4.) Potential headache sources must be considered efficiently.

Table 2.4 is a suggested list of laboratory analyses. A complete chemistry profile, complete blood count (CBC), endocrinological tests, and urinalysis should be obtained in all patients with troublesome headache conditions. (These factors also assist in determining the baseline values necessary to safely administer pharmacotherapy for headache.)

Urine and blood drug evaluations are used for detecting the presence of unsuspected medication/drugs, toxic amounts of known medication, and general safety parameters for the implementation of pharmacotherapy. *Patients may not report their use (or excessive use) of over-the-counter or prescribed analgesics, tranquilizers, or other medications or drugs that are relevant to both the origin of headache or to the safety of planned pharmacotherapy.*

IV. Standard Neurodiagnostic Studies

In general, we believe that most patients with headache will require neurodiagnostic testing. A CT scan or MRI should be performed in most patients with headaches severe enough to prompt medical evaluation and treatment. An exception may be occasional and infrequent headaches, or those that are specifi-

---

TABLE 2.4. **SELECTED INITIAL LABORATORY EVALUATION**

BUN[a]	CBC[a]
Creatinine	ESR[a]
SGOT[a]	Serum B_{12}
SGPT[a]	Folate
Alkaline phosphatase	Serum estrogen (females)
Total bilirubin	Free T_4
Total protein	TSH
Albumin	Urinalysis
Calcium	Urine drug screen
Phosphorus	
Sodium	
Potassium	
Glucose	
Triglycerides	
Cholesterol	
HDL[a] cholesterol	

[a]BUN, blood urea nitrogen; SGOT, serum glutamic oxaloacetic transaminase; SGPT, serum glutamic pyruvic transaminase; HDL, high-density lipoprotein; CBC, complete blood count; TSH, thyroid stimulating hormone; erythrocyte sedimentation rate.

cally and only associated with menstruation and are otherwise characteristic of migraine.

A. Computerized Tomographic (CT) Scan

A CT scan of the brain and head is indicated to rule out structural disease, such as tumor, abscess, hydrocephalus, stroke, and hemorrhage. It is particularly important whenever there are neurological or mental symptoms or findings and in the presence of persistent or recurring headache, not easily and effectively managed by standard medication.

Even when the headache is well managed, a CT (or MRI) scan may nonetheless be prudent. Many analgesics and preventive medications can relieve or mask headache associated with organic disease. Subdural hematomas, obstructive syndromes, and A-V malformations, among others, can mimic the primary headache conditions or activate migraine (a point deserving repetition) and at least initially respond to standard headache treatment.

Moreover, migraine, appropriately treated with standard therapy, is occasionally accompanied by a second (often silent at first) illness or other organic process, which cannot be distinguished from migraine clinically.

B. Magnetic Resonance Imaging (MRI)

An MRI of the head, and perhaps of the cervical spine and neck, is indicated for many of the same reasons as the CT scan. The MRI should be ordered instead of or in addition to the CT scan in order to:

1. Identify lesions in the brainstem and occipital-cervical junction that are not well visualized by CT scanning; such as Arnold-Chiari malformation, cervical disc disease, and spondylosis.
2. Visualize the pituitary region better than can be achieved with CT scanning;
3. Avoid contrast material, as in a contrast-enhanced CT scan. (A contrast MRI [see below] can be beneficial but may not be essential in some instances.);
4. Rule out demyelinating, ischemic, or inflammatory disease;
5. Evaluate carotid and anterior neck soft tissue (carotodynia, suspected carotid dissection, etc.)—(see MRI angiogram); and
6. Evaluate facial and retropharyngeal regions.

While the cost of MRI is considerably more than that of the CT scan, *clinical judgment must prevail, and cost con-*

siderations should not compromise clinical opinion. MRI is rapidly becoming the standard diagnostic test for intracranial disease. In the presence of resistant or difficult cases of head or face pain, it must be performed and expertly interpreted.

Employing gadolinium enhances the MRI and increases signal intensity and may be particularly valuable in visualizing suspected tumors, for example.

MRI angiography (MRA) has not yet inspired the level of confidence of arteriography in evaluation of aneurysm and vasculitis, and should not be considered a substitute. However, MRA does provide a means by which vascular anatomy can be evaluated without apparent risk or discomfort (noninvasive). It may have particular value in evaluating cervical vascular disease, including dissection of the carotid artery.

MRI is currently considered a safe procedure. However, pregnant women, particularly during the first and second trimester, should not undergo MRI because of the concern that magnetic fields and radio waves may impose an adverse influence on the unborn fetus.

C. The Lumbar Puncture (LP)

The conditions that can be identified only or most conclusively by evaluation of cerebrospinal fluid (CSF) include:

1. Elevation or reduction in cerebral spinal fluid pressure; and
2. Bleeding and/or infection, inflammation, or cellular infiltration (lymphoma, etc.) in the central nervous system.

The indications for an LP and CSF evaluation are listed in Table 2.5.

The LP should not be performed until CT scan or MRI has ruled out the presence of intracranial structural disease, which could induce unforeseeable risk were an LP to be undertaken. The one exception might be the urgent need to evaluate the CSF when there is strong suspicion of a rapidly pro-

---

TABLE 2.5. **INDICATIONS FOR LP AND CSF EVALUATION**

1. Abrupt and sudden onset of headache;
2. Headache accompanied by signs or symptoms of infection (fever, stiff neck, etc.);
3. Suspicion of bleeding or infiltrative/inflammatory processes;
4. Suspicion of elevated or reduced pressure, often indicated by a postural component to the headache; and
5. Headache attacks associated with cranial nerve deficits that could result from infiltrative, tumor, or infectious involvement of the brainstem.

gressive infectious disorder and a CT scan or MRI is not readily available.

In the presence of acute sudden-onset headache, sufficient to raise concern regarding the possible presence of intracranial hemorrhage, a CT scan (first with and then without contrast) should be performed, followed by an LP, and done within the first 48 hours to rule out a subarachnoid hemorrhage. *The absence of blood on CSF evaluation does not in itself eliminate the possibility of subarachnoid hemorrhage, since blood may not enter the spinal canal for several hours after hemorrhage.* However, delaying the LP for days or longer allows the blood to be resorbed, sometimes without a trace, although xanthochromic CSF fluid is generally evident for at least a week following hemorrhage.

The CSF must be handled properly. At least two tubes must be evaluated for cellular components, thereby providing a comparative measurement. We suggest a cell count for tubes 2 and 4. Cerebrospinal fluid must be analyzed soon after it is obtained. The CSF must also be centrifuged immediately if discoloration is present or if there is a suspicion of blood, in order to assess for the presence of xanthochromia. If blood cells are allowed to remain for long in the spinal fluid tubes prior to processing, lysis may occur and the fluid may become xanthochromic, thereby complicating the interpretation.

Accurate opening and closing pressures must be documented. Closing pressure is of particular value in cases of pseudotumor cerebri (benign intracranial pressure) to determine if severe lowering of CSF pressure occurs with minimal fluid removal.

D. Electroencephalography (EEG)

The EEG assists in evaluating:

1. Paroxysmal electrical activity, indicating a predisposition to seizure activity; and
2. Neuronal disturbances resulting from drug or metabolic illness and primary neurological disease.

The EEG is particularly important in the presence of periodic or continuous mental changes, such as confusion, memory impairment, amnesia, and personality change. Baseline EEG studies are important to determine paroxysmal EEG activity that might indicate an increased seizure tendency when the patient is placed on certain headache medications. Many lower the seizure threshold, such as antidepressants and phenothiazines. Just as cardiac function must be monitored carefully during treatment with drugs that influence cardiac rhythm and rate (see below), the same is true when using drugs that affect cerebral function.

Some authorities believe that recurring headache in the presence of distinct paroxysmal EEG patterns may be particularly responsive to anticonvulsant therapy.

E. Electrocardiography (ECG)

Most medications used in the pharmacological treatment of headache can affect heart function, rhythm, and rate or blood pressure, including the antidepressants, β-blockers, calcium channel blockers, and others. Therefore, establishing a baseline ECG prior to the implementation of these treatments is prudent and medically protective. Rarely, primary cardiac disease, such as periodic arrhythmias resulting in ischemia, is related to the cause of headache.

F. Routine X-rays

Cervical spine and skull x-rays may be indicated in specific circumstances, such as in suspected fracture, bone disease, etc.

G. Arteriography/MRI Angiography (MRA)

These studies are generally not routinely required in the evaluation of head pain syndromes. They are indicated, however, when there is a strong suspicion of aneurysm, vasculitis, stroke, or other condition that can be evaluated only by the study of cervical and cerebral circulation. (MRI angiography is not yet established as an entirely reliable test for these circumstances, but growing reliance is apparent in centers with advanced experience and technique.)

H. Ultrasound Testing

Ultrasound evaluation of the carotid vascular system and heart may be indicated to:

1. Evaluate the carotid arteries and the heart in cases of headache accompanied by periodic neurological events associated with headache; and
2. Evaluate carotid artery flow dynamics.

The value of transcranial Doppler evaluation in the diagnosis of cerebral flow patterns is still controversial.

I. Evoked Response Testing

Sensory, auditory, or visual evoked response testing may have a role in a variety of neurological conditions associated with headache, including *post-concussion syndrome* (brainstem auditory evoked response), headache in the presence of significant visual disturbances (visual evoked response), and headache associated with various sensory symptoms (somatosensory evoked response). Visual evoked responses can assist in evaluating and monitoring the progression of visual disturbances in pseudotumor cerebri (see Chapter 16).

V. Other Evaluations
A. Temporomandibular Joint (TMJ) and Dental Evaluations

The jaw and dental structures may be important in headache and face pain conditions. Underlying migraine may be exacerbated, or a new headache can develop as a direct result of dental disease or procedures, such as root canal or extractions, and in the presence of significant malocclusion. Jaw and occlusive disease can generally be identified by aggravation of pain upon chewing, jaw opening, and related motions (see Chapter 11).

Microabscesses subsequent to tooth extraction, or neuromas secondary to root canal may produce chronic head or facial pain. Surgical procedures that interrupt the dental nerves may result in neuronal disturbances within the *nucleus caudalis* of the *fifth cranial nerve* in the brainstem. Disruption in the trigeminal system, so closely related to the important pain modulating systems of the brainstem (see Chapter 3), may explain an unexpected onset of head and facial pain following dental procedures.

Temporomandibular joint (TMJ) dysfunction, often overstated and overtreated as a cause of headache and facial pain, can nonetheless be important in some instances. The pain can arise from the joint itself, the surrounding soft tissue, or the muscles.

MRI of the temporomandibular joints is primarily useful in assessing degenerative disease or displacement within the joint itself and is indicated in selected circumstances. We recommend referral to a qualified dental professional who understands headache and face pain and shares a conservative and prudent view toward the treatment of jaw disorders.

B. Selected Tests to Evaluate for Suspected Stroke or Vasculitis

Recently, increased attention has focused on the possible risk of stroke in certain patients with headache who experience periodic neurological events. The presence of anticardiolipin antibodies, lupus anticoagulant, and other clotting abnormalities might predispose to stroke-like events. Table 2.6 provides a recommended (selected) laboratory diagnostic battery for assessing stroke risk in patients with significant periodic neurological events and headache, and which should be evaluated in conjunction with neurodiagnostic testing.

Coagulation abnormalities are important, and recent evidence suggests that inherited deficiencies of antithrombin III, protein C, and protein S are associated with arterial and venous occlusive brain infarction. These studies, in conjunction with a careful neurological examination and neurodiagnostic assessment, including carotid ultrasound, MRI of the brain (? MRI angiogram), echocardiogram, and Holter cardiac monitoring, are indicated when significant periodic neurological events (other than simple visual auras) are present in patients with headache. They are indicated in the presence of *complicated migraine*. Complicated migraine is characterized

---

TABLE 2.6. **LABORATORY EVALUATION FOR ASSESSING STROKE RISK IN HEADACHE PATIENTS**

Hemoglobin, hematocrit, and platelet count
Anticardiolipin antibodies (see Levine, 1991 and Iniguez, 1991 in Chapter 7)
Lupus anticoagulant
Antinuclear antibody (ANA)
Double and single-stranded anti-DNA antibodies (if ANA-positive)
Complement levels
Rheumatoid factor
Sedimentation rate
Serum protein electrophoresis
Fasting lipid profile, glucose

TABLE 2.7. **SELECTED INVESTIGATIONS FOR HEAD, NECK, AND FACE PAIN**

History and physical examination (including neurological exam)
Laboratory evaluation (see text)
CT scan
MRI and MRA
Electroencephalography
Lumbar puncture/CSF evaluation
Ultrasound studies
Cardiac evaluation
Dental/jaw evaluation
Diagnostic blockade
EMG of cervical musculature
Myelogram
Arteriography
Evoked response tests
Otolaryngological evaluation
Ophthalmological evaluation

by a prolonged neurological event, which may outlast the headache by hours or days, or a migraine that is associated with transient intense neurological deficits. The use of oral contraceptives and estrogens and the presence of smoking are considered additional risk factors for stroke.

C. Diagnostic Blocks

Diagnostic blocking of structures such as the occipital nerve, C2–C3 facet joints and nerves, supraorbital nerve, sphenopalatine ganglia, the styloid process, or stylomandibular ligament (see Chapters 11 and 17) may provide important clues to diagnosis and offer specific treatment interventions as well.

Establishing a definitive diagnosis based solely upon the value of any of the blocking procedures is tenuous, as these procedures are known to relieve pain in a variety of conditions not directly related to the targeted structure. The blocked nerves or ganglia are often involved in the transmission of pain impulses from a number of sources, and effective blocking may not itself constitute the basis for a reliable diagnosis.

Summary

Recurring head, neck, and face pain must be evaluated with the same intensity, completeness, and objectivity as that accorded to other important clinical conditions. The diagnosis of migraine or other primary headache disorder cannot be made without consideration and perhaps exclusion of certain conditions that can mimic, accompany, or activate primary headache syndromes. Invasive testing can usually be avoided, but the occasional need for these cannot be overlooked. Table 2.7 lists selected investigations for head, neck, and face pain evaluation.

Diagnostic testing should not replace a comprehensive history and physical examination, but a history and physical examination cannot substitute for adequate laboratory and diagnostic testing.

3

Mechanisms and Theories of Head Pain

I. Introduction

The precise origins of recurring, benign (chronic) head pain have not yet been established, but important advances have been made in the past decade. There is increasing support for the concept that benign recurring head pain originates in the structures of the brain, specifically neurons and ascending/descending projection systems within the brainstem. Disturbances of neurotransmitter/receptor function and neurovascular control and inflammation are the focus of much current research.

What follows is a brief and selected review of specific concepts regarding the mechanisms of headache, particularly migraine. It is not intended to be an all-encompassing study of the topic. The reader is directed to more extensive reviews (see references) for further discussion.

II. Anatomical Considerations

A. Pain-Sensitive Structures

Pain-sensitive intracranial structures include the skin and blood vessels of the scalp, the head and neck muscles (see Chapter 17 for a more extensive discussion of neck structures), the venous sinuses, the arteries of the meninges, the larger cerebral arteries, the pain-carrying fibers of the fifth, ninth, and tenth cranial nerves, and parts of the dura mater at the base of the brain. The brain itself is insensitive to pain.

B. Pain Pathways

In general, pain is transmitted from the periphery by *small myelinated (α-δ) fibers* (sharp pain) and *unmyelinated c-fibers* (aching, burning pain) which terminate in the dorsal horn of the spinal cord. Secondary neurons from the dorsal horn reach the thalamus via the spinal thalamic pathways.

Substance P, a neuropeptide, may be the pain neurotransmitter for the primary sensory neurons. Interneurons in the dorsal horn use *enkephalins* and perhaps *γ-aminobutyric acid (GABA)* as an inhibitory neurotransmitter to block pain transmission.

Figure 3.1 illustrates the pain fiber pathways transmitting pain from the face, head, and neck regions. The upper cer-

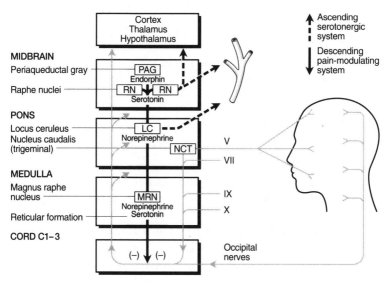

Figure 3.1. Pain pathways.

vical spinal cord contains pain fiber systems for the entire head and neck region.

1. Ascending pain pathways

The neothalamic pathway (quality of pain) terminates in the ventrobasal nucleus of the thalamus, which projects to the somatosensory cortex. The paleothalamic pathway (emotional content of pain) sends projections to the reticular formation of the brainstem, the periaqueductal gray, the hypothalamic, and the medial and intralaminar thalamic nuclei.

Within the brainstem is an *ascending serotonergic system* that originates in the midbrain raphe region, innervates the cerebral blood vessels, and is distributed to the thalamus, hypothalamus, and cortex. The neurons of this system appear to be involved in cerebral blood flow, sleep, and neuroendocrine control, among other influences.

2. Descending pain-modulating system

The *descending pain-modulating system* originates in the *periaqueductal gray (PAG)* in the midbrain and synapses in the raphe magnus in the medulla, and from there connects to the spinal tract of the trigeminal nerve and the dorsal horn of the first, second, and third cervical roots in the spinal cord. Norepinephrine, serotonin, and opiates mediate this important system that modulates (inhibits) pain transmission from most regions of the head and neck.

Thus, within this brainstem and spinal cord there exists a system to carry pain to the thalamus and cortex and a system to modulate pain or inhibit it (the pain-modulating system).

III. Physiological Considerations
A. Pain Mechanisms

Head pain is mediated in part by the first division of the trigeminal nerve. Pain fibers descend in the brainstem and converge on cells in the posterior horn of the upper cervical spinal cord, which also receive input from the upper cervical sensory roots, as well as other sources. Head pain arising from organic causes can be the result of traction, displacement, inflammation, or pressure on nociceptors in pain-sensitive structures. Nociceptor information is then relayed to the brainstem and spinal cord. Peripheral activation of nociceptors alone, however, is not likely to be the primary cause of migraine or muscle-type headaches. Quite possibly, pain can be generated by *a primary dysfunction of central ascending and/or descending pain-related systems and involve input from supraspinal, vascular, and myogenic sources* (see Olesen, 1991).

B. Neurogenic Inflammation

Neural connections exist between the trigeminal nerve and intracranial blood vessels. Substance P, calcitonin gene-related peptide (CGRP), and neurokinin A (NKA) are located in the trigeminal sensory neurons, which innervate the cephalic blood vessels.

Stimulation of these nerves results in the peripheral release of neuropeptides, including substance P, producing neurogenic inflammation with increased vascular permeability, dilation of blood vessels, plasma extravasation, and platelet injury.

Migraine and cluster headache have traditionally been called "vascular headaches" because of the recognized involvement of blood vessels. Initially, the blood vessels and ischemic or vasodilatory changes were considered to be the primary mechanism by which pain or neurological symptoms occurred. It is now believed that constriction or dilation phenomena may be *incidental* to events taking place in the trigeminal vascular neurons originating in the brainstem.

It is not currently known whether the neurogenic inflammation is the primary mechanism of head pain. The intracranial release of substance P and CGRP may explain why dilation of intracranial vessels may be accompanied by pain, as in migraine, but not under normal physiological circumstances such as physical exertion or a hot bath. CGRP is, in fact, released in the jugular venous blood during an attack of migraine.

The antimigraine drugs ergotamine tartrate and sumatriptan (a 5-HT_1 receptor agonist) prevent neurogenic-induced inflammation in the rat dura mater by blocking neurotransmission in small myelinated C-fibers peripherally or within the brain itself. This action appears unrelated to constriction of the blood vessels, no longer thought to be a primary mechanism by which so-called vasoconstrictive antimigraine medications work.

IV. Traditional Concepts in Headache Pathogenesis
A. The "Muscle Theory"
The muscular contraction (tension) concept of headache states that tension-type headaches are secondary to increased muscle contraction in the pericranial and cervical musculature. Studies, however, do not support this mechanism as a primary cause of pain. In fact, more muscle contraction is present in migraineurs than in tension headache patients!

B. The "Vascular Theory" of Migraine
This concept is fundamentally committed to the belief that migraine aura is primarily due to cerebral ischemia from vasoconstriction as the initial event and that the headache itself is the result of reactive vasodilation. Pain is thought to be enhanced by vasoactive polypeptides in the tissues surrounding the external carotid artery.

However, cerebral blood flow (CBF) studies do not support the traditional vascular theory. A decrease in CBF does occur during migraine with aura, but not in migraine without aura. Moreover, *the changes in migraine with aura are not sufficient nor anatomically consistent to explain the neurological events.*

In migraine with aura, a wave of reduced blood flow (oligemia) spreads forward from the occipital area and precedes the aura. It persists into the headache phase.

Historically important work by Leão demonstrated that electrically stimulated rabbit cortex exhibited a wave of *spreading electrical depression* that moved over the cortex at a rate of 2–3 mm/minute. This rate of *spreading depression* is similar to the spread of oligemia (reduced blood flow) in patients with *migraine with aura*.

Lashley, a researcher who himself suffered migraine with aura, mapped out the rate of progression of his own scintillating scotoma across his visual field. He calculated that it corresponded to a rate over his occipital cortex of 2–3 mm/minute.

Thus, the rate of development of the scotomata, spreading oligemia, and spreading electrical depression are approximately the same. Many authorities now believe that the oligemia is secondary to a primary neurogenic event.

IV. The Neurogenic Concepts

The neurogenic theory of migraine suggests that migraine is caused by a primary disturbance of brain function. Cerebral blood flow studies in migraine with aura are most consistent with a primary neuronal event producing secondary vascular changes. Magnetoencephalographic studies of the brain during a migraine attack support the concept of spreading depression in migraine, as described above.

In favor of the neurogenic concept of migraine are:

- The presence of premonitory symptoms suggestive of hypothalamic origin;
- The visual aura that crosses vascular territories (due to spreading depression?);
- Associated symptoms, such as nausea/vomiting, and hypersensitivity to sensory stimuli;
- Magnetoencephalographic findings confirming spreading depression; and
- Magnetic resonance spectroscopy showing increased high-energy phosphate consumption and low intracellular magnesium.

These studies and the data described below suggest that the brain of migraineurs, even between attacks, is physiologically abnormal (see Welch, 1990).

A. Serotonin Considerations

Serotonin, 5-hydroxytryptamine (5-HT), is widely distributed throughout the body. Major concentrations occur in the gastrointestinal tract (90%), the platelets (8%), and the brain. Blood serotonin, which is mainly in the platelets, falls at the time of a migraine attack but is normal between attacks. A low molecular weight platelet serotonin-releasing factor has been identified in the blood only during migraine attacks.

Moreover, platelet serotonin content is low in patients with chronic tension-type headaches, which may support the concept that the tension-type headache is a variant of migraine.

A relationship between serotonin and migraine is further suggested by the observation that migraine can be precipitated by reserpine (a serotonin-depleting agent) and relieved by serotonin and serotonin agonists.

B. Serotonin Receptors

There are at least four classes of 5-HT receptors: 5-HT_1, 5-HT_2, 5-HT_3, and 5-HT_4, with subtypes of these classes. All have been identified in the brain. The 5-HT_1 and 5-HT_2 receptors are influenced by estrogen. Aging results in a decrease in serotonin receptors and generally an improvement in migraine. The 5-HT_1 receptors are most dense in the hippocampus, the dorsal raphe, and the substantia nigra, with lesser concentrations in the cortex. 5-HT_1 receptors are inhibitory, while 5-HT_2, 5-HT_3, and 5-HT_4 receptors are excitatory.

In humans, there are at least three 5-HT_1 receptor subtypes—5-HT_{1a}, 5-HT_{1c}, and 5-HT_{1d}. Stimulation of the 5-HT_{1a} receptor is implicated in anxiety mechanisms.

The 5-HT_{1d} receptor is the most widespread serotonin receptor in the brain and functions as an autoreceptor modulating neurotransmitter release. Receptor activation inhibits release of 5-HT, norepinephrine, and acetylcholine and substance P.

Moreover, 5-HT_{1d} receptors are found on cerebral blood vessels. Stimulation results in closure of A-V shunts in dogs and cats and appears to produce vasoconstriction, bronchoconstriction, gastrointestinal smooth muscle contraction, and platelet aggregation.

V. Tentative Concepts on the Pharmacology of Antimigraine Drugs

Many of the drugs which are effective in migraine are believed to affect one or more of the various serotonin receptors. Methysergide, cyproheptadine, dihydroergotamine (DHE), tricyclic antidepressants, and verapamil interact with the 5-HT_2 receptor. β-propanolol, sumatriptan, and DHE interact at the 5-HT_{1a} receptor, while sumatriptan and DHE work at the 5-HT_{1d} receptor as well.

DHE and sumatriptan block neurogenic inflammation, and both may help in the modulation of the central serotonin pain system.

Thus, while the traditional view of headache pathogenesis relies upon explanations involving vasoconstriction, vasodilation, and muscle relaxation, increasing data support the view that neurogenic concepts are of primary importance. Moreover, most drugs that control migraine preventively, and perhaps symptomatically as well, appear to do so via a mechanism involving serotonin or serotonin receptor dynamics.

4

Differential Diagnosis of Headache

I. Introduction

Over 300 entities cause headache. The *primary headache disorders*, such as migraine, and cluster headache, are those in which headache represents the primary symptom or at least one of the primary symptoms of a basic physiological disorder. These disorders are absent of definable, pathological abnormalities. The primary headache conditions generally but not exclusively reflect an inherited biological predisposition.

The *secondary headache conditions* are those in which the headache represents a symptom of a pathological, organic process. Table 4.1 lists selected general categories of illness that can produce secondary headaches (See also Chapter 11).

A headache differential diagnosis can be approached in several ways, though admittedly none is entirely satisfactory. We have chosen to approach headache from a temporal perspective, that is, certain conditions produce headache with a characteristic pattern of onset and evolution. Some are explosive and sudden in onset. Others begin insidiously or subacutely and progress in intensity and frequency.

This chapter reviews the key differential diagnostic possibilities within the context of three temporal patterns of headache. Because many of the conditions demonstrate more than one temporal pattern, conditions may be listed in more than one category.

Clearly, assignment to a category is arbitrary, and an astute awareness of most of the diagnostic possibilities is required.

The three temporal categories include:

1. Sudden, abrupt-onset headache;
2. Intermittent, recurrent headache; and
3. Subacute, persistent, progressive headache.

II. Sudden-Onset, Rapidly Worsening, Severe Headache ("First or Worst" Syndrome)
A. Description

A sudden-onset, "first or worst" headache must always be assumed to be the result of an acute neurological event, although frequently it reflects nothing more than a severe migraine or cluster attack. Changes in awareness or cognition,

TABLE 4.1. **SELECTED CATEGORIES OF ILLNESSES THAT CAUSE HEADACHE**

Intracranial structural disease
Infectious disease (including AIDS, sinusitis, etc.)
Cerebrovascular ischemia
Cerebral vein thrombosis
Metabolic disease
Toxic exposures
Primary headache conditions
Central nervous system pressure disorders (high and low)
Vasculitis and collagen vascular disease
Hemorrhage (parenchymal and subarachnoid)
Traumatic conditions
Withdrawal syndromes
Severe hypertension
Dental, cranial vault, temporomandibular joint, and myofascial disease
Cervical spine and occipitocervical junction disease

or the presence of neurological signs or symptoms, suggest but do not in themselves establish with certainty the presence of an intracranial or systemic process.

Central nervous system (CNS) organic disease can provoke what would otherwise appear to be typical migraine attacks. A rapid-onset, severe migraine may be difficult to differentiate from the symptoms of a subarachnoid hemorrhage (SAH).

Among the key and worrisome features of a sudden, severe, rapidly worsening headache are:

1. Abrupt-onset (unexpected event) that rapidly progresses in seconds to minutes;
2. Accompaniments, which may include nausea and vomiting, fever, stiff neck, focal neurological findings, papilledema, changes in mental function or level of consciousness, among others;
3. A continuing, persistent, or progressive pattern, even though in some serious circumstances, the pain may abate somewhat.

Table 4.2 lists selected diagnostic possibilities characterized by sudden-onset severe headache.

B. Selected Topics

1. Subarachnoid hemorrhage (SAH)

Subarachnoid hemorrhage (SAH) from a ruptured aneurysm occurs in 28,000 people per year in North America. It typically presents as an acute-, sudden-onset, bilateral severe headache (often called "thunderclap headache") associated with nuchal rigidity (within 24 hours), photopho-

TABLE 4.2. **CONDITIONS ASSOCIATED WITH SUDDEN-ONSET HEADACHE**

Subarachnoid hemorrhage (aneurysm or arteriovenous malformation)
Brain hemorrhage
Acute subdural or epidural hematoma
Acute severe hypertension
  Pressor response
  Pheochromocytoma
  Malignant hypertension
Acute glaucoma
Internal carotid dissection or other acute carotid syndromes
Acute obstructive disease (from tumor, etc.)
Head trauma (hemorrhage, cavernous sinus thrombosis, etc.) (See Chapter 12)

The following conditions may cause sudden-onset attacks but are more likely to
  be subacute in presentation.
Encephalitis/meningitis
Sinusitis/periorbital cellulitis
Cerebral vein thrombosis
Optic neuritis
Migraine
Ischemic cerebrovascular disease
Cerebral vasculitis

bia, nausea, vomiting, and perhaps obtundation or coma.
The *sentinel headache* is a severe sudden-onset headache
that represents a warning of impending catastrophic hemorrhage and occurs prior to this event. The *sentinel headache* may manifest as a severe headache alone or in association with nausea, vomiting, and, occasionally, stiff
neck. It is not easily distinguished from an acute migraine,
and in a person with a history of migraine, it may not be
distinguishable at all.

Subarachnoid hemorrhage from an arteriovenous (A-V)
malformation may be less dramatic than from an aneurysm.

If headache is suspected to be associated with frank subarachnoid hemorrhage or impending hemorrhage, an extensive neurological evaluation is necessary, including a
CT scan (with and without contrast) and lumbar puncture
(LP). The value of MRI or MR angiography (MRA) to rule
out an aneurysm is currently tenuous. The need for arteriography in suspected cases must be determined on an individual basis. Most authorities believe that if a CT scan
(with and without contrast) and an LP are normal within
24 hours of the attack, further invasive studies, such as
arteriography, are not necessary. There are, however,
noteworthy exceptions, such as the case of Day and Raskin

(1986) in which the authors describe three acute-onset (sentinel) headaches, the first two of which were associated with normal CT scan and lumbar puncture. The third attack prompted arteriography, which demonstrated an aneurysm.

2. Spontaneous, acute brain (parenchymal) hemorrhage

Cerebral or cerebellar hemorrhage has been reported to occur in patients with migraine, with and without previous hypertension. Whether migraine is itself a risk factor to hemorrhage remains uncertain. Unlike subarachnoid hemorrhage, acute parenchymal hemorrhage is more likely associated with acute neurological signs. Distinguishing the headache due to parenchymal hemorrhage from that of subarachnoid hemorrhage may be difficult if blood enters the ventricular system and if neurological events are present. Parenchymal hemorrhage can also result from bleeding into a brain tumor.

3. Acute, severe hypertension

Suddenly elevated hypertension (greater than 25% rise in diastolic pressure or a combined pressure of 180/130 mm Hg) can produce a severe, sudden-onset headache. More moderate elevations of systolic and/or diastolic pressure, though frequent accompaniments of migraine, do not cause headache. Stupor, seizures, or focal neurological signs are present in *hypertensive encephalopathy*. Pressor responses result from toxic or medication effects (e.g., monoamine oxidase inhibitor (MAOI) etc.). *Pheochromocytoma* is associated with diaphoresis, palpitations, and anxiety symptomatology and is diagnosed by chemical and imaging tests (see II. B. 5., below).

4. Acute angle closure glaucoma

Glaucoma often presents with sudden-onset orbital and eye pain associated with headache, pupillary changes conjunctival injection, lens clouding, and sometimes nausea, vomiting, and other symptoms. The demonstration of elevated intraocular pressure is diagnostic. *Onset may occur following the use of anticholinergic drugs.* Tables 4.3 and 4.4 list the ocular and otolaryngological causes of headache. (See Chapter 11 for the differential diagnosis of causes of face pain.)

5. Spontaneous internal carotid artery dissection

Spontaneous dissection of the carotid artery is an uncommon but important cause of sudden-onset headache and

TABLE 4.3. **SELECTED OCULAR CATEGORIES OF HEADACHE (SEE CHAPTER 11 FOR ADDITIONAL LISTINGS)**

Glaucoma
  Narrow angle glaucoma
  Neovascular glaucoma (from neovascularization secondary to disease, such as carotid stenosis, retinal vein or artery occlusion, diabetic retinopathy, etc.)
Corneal and conjunctival disease
Asthenopia
Retrobulbar neuritis
Ischemic ocular inflammation
Uveitis (intraocular inflammatory disease)
Diseases of the orbit
  Cellulitis
  Inflammatory or noninflammatory orbital pseudotumor
  Orbital myositis
  Lacrimal gland disease (tumors, cysts, infection)
  Posterior scleritis
Herpes zoster ophthalmicus
Painful ophthalmoplegia (Tolosa-Hunt syndrome)
Cavernous sinus thrombosis, fistula, aneurysm

TABLE 4.4. **SELECTED OTOLARYNGOLOGICAL CATEGORIES OF HEADACHE (SEE CHAPTER 11 FOR ADDITIONAL LISTINGS)**

Cerumen impaction
External otitis
Herpes zoster oticus
Myringitis (tympanic membrane inflammation)
Otitis media
Mastoiditis
Gradenigo syndrome (CN VI palsy, eye pain, and sometimes discharge from the ear) from temporal bone infection (petrositis)
Eagle's syndrome (elongation of the styloid process)
Ernest syndrome (stylomandibular ligament syndrome)
Carotidynia
Temporomandibular joint syndrome
Cranial neuralgias (glossopharyngeal neuralgia, superior laryngeal neuralgia)
Malignancy (primary and metastatic), infiltrative, nasopharyngeal cancer, etc.
Denture misfittings
Nasal disease/septum deformities
Sinus disease
  Infectious, granulomatous, abscess
  Occlusive/obstructive
Others

acute neurological symptoms. The headache is often unilateral and located in the orbital, periorbital, frontal, or neck regions. Stroke-related symptoms and pupillary changes (including a Horner's syndrome) can accompany or precede the headache. Internal carotid artery dissection should be considered in the presence of acute-onset headache or neck pain, pupillary disturbance or Horner's syndrome, tinnitus, and the presence of stroke-like symptoms. Magnetic resonance angiography of the neck and carotid arteriography are the diagnostic interventions most frequently used.

Giant cell arteritis, atherosclerotic thrombosis, fibromuscular dysplasia, and carotid aneurysm, as well as parenchymal brain hemorrhage, may produce a similar clinical picture. (See Chapter 13 for further discussion of spontaneous internal carotid artery dissection.)

III. Subacute, Intermittent, Recurrent Headaches
A. Description

Awareness of the existence of previous similar headache attacks is helpful in placing subsequent attacks into the proper diagnostic perspective. Table 4.5 lists illnesses capable of producing a subacute onset and recurring headache.

B. Selected Topics
1. A-V malformation

A-V malformation may present with acute, sudden-onset subarachnoid hemorrhage or with episodic bouts of migraine-like headache, sometimes preceded by neurological symptoms typical of *migraine with aura*.

TABLE 4.5. **CONDITIONS ASSOCIATED WITH SUBACUTE-ONSET AND RECURRING, INTERMITTENT HEADACHE**

Cerebrovascular ischemia (TIA, embolic disease, etc.)
Cerebral vein thrombosis, including cavernous sinus thrombosis, fistula, etc.
Obstructive hydrocephalus, including Arnold-Chiari malformation type I
Pheochromocytoma
Neuralgic syndromes
Cluster headache, chronic paroxysmal hemicrania
Migraine
Cerebral vasculitis
Cerebral tumors (most commonly a progressive, worsening course, but can be
   intermittent initially)
Benign idiopathic intracranial hypertension (pseudotumor cerebri)
Recurring hemorrhage from A-V malformation
Sentinel headache
Headache associated with substances or their withdrawal (ergotamine, caffeine,
   narcotics, etc.)
Subdural hematoma (usually progressive, but can be intermittent)
Occipitocervical junction disease
CSF hypotension
Dental, cranial vault, TM joint disease
Cranial, paranasal sinusitis (see Druce, 1991; see Chapter 11)

2. Cerebral ischemia

Cerebral ischemia and stroke may result in continuing or episodic headaches that may precede, accompany, or follow the acute neurological event. Neurological symptomatology is usually evident within 48 hours of headache onset, but not always. Approximately 35% of patients with stroke present with headache, and 25% of patients with a transient ischemic attack (TIA) experience headache. The headache is nonspecific. Clinical differentiation between embolic, thrombotic, and hemorrhagic disease is often impossible on clinical grounds. Table 4.6 lists the cerebrovascular causes of headache.

3. Cerebral vein thrombosis

Thrombotic occlusion of the dural sinus and cerebral veins can produce severe intermittent or continuous headache. Thrombosis of the sagittal sinus can result in headache, intracranial hypertension with papilledema, focal neurological seizures, and if hemorrhagic infarction occurs, progressive obtundation.

Cavernous sinus thrombosis causes pain around the eye and over the forehead, together with conjunctival changes, proptosis, ophthalmoplegia, and occasionally edema of the face.

For venous thrombotic syndromes, contrast CT scanning, MRI, MRA, and/or arteriography are important diagnostic interventions, as are appropriate laboratory studies to rule out coagulopathic illness.

Treatment of cerebral vein thrombosis includes reduction of intracranial pressure, anticoagulation, and treatment

---

TABLE 4.6.   **CEREBROVASCULAR DISEASES CAUSING HEADACHE**

Occlusive vascular disease
   Transient ischemic attack (TIA)
   Internal carotid artery occlusion or stenosis
   Occlusion of middle cerebral artery
   Vertebral basilar occlusion
   Thrombosis of cerebral veins or dural sinus
   Fibromuscular hyperplasia
   Embolic disease
   Vasculitis
Hypertension
Hemorrhage
   Subarachnoid hemorrhage
   Cerebellar/cerebral parenchymal hemorrhage
   Subdural and epidural hematoma

of seizures, if present. Headache may improve with reso-
lution of the condition but may prove resistant to early
treatment, other than with narcotic analgesics. Patients may
present with features similar to those of pseudotumor cerebri (benign increased intracranial pressure; see later and
Chapter 16), particularly when there is involvement of the
lateral sinus (*otitic hydrocephalus*).

4. Obstructive hydrocephalus

Obstructive hydrocephalus may produce headache with
gait disturbances, changes in cognition, or other neurological events. Postural abnormalities, worsened by exertion
or neck posture, are noted frequently. Enlargement of the
ventricular system, as seen by CT scanning, and increased
intracranial pressure are diagnostic features. Headache is
usually improved with reduction in pressure. Intermittent
elevations result in periodic headaches.

5. Pheochromocytoma

Pheochromocytoma can produce episodic headache, often
provoked by exertion or from certain medications such as
β-adrenergic blocking agents. Periodic or sustained elevations of blood pressure, excessive perspiration, and palpitations and anxiety symptoms are usually present. A family history is noted in approximately 10% of cases. This
disorder can be associated with *neurofibromatosis* and *café
au lait spots*. The diagnosis of pheochromocytoma is based
largely on biochemical evidence, including elevated urinary catecholamines and related metabolites (metane-
phrine, normetanephrine, and vanillylmandelic acid) from
a 24-hour urine specimen, as well as CT localization of the
abdominal tumor.

6. Systemic or intracranial infection

Systemic or intracranial infection can produce severe
headache. Alternately, severe migraine or migraine-like
headaches may be activated by systemic or CNS infection.
The presence of fever or signs of infection accompanying
headache mandates a complete evaluation. A stiff neck may
or may not be present. Photophobia is common. (See page
33 for further discussion.) In most instances, infection produces a progressive or persistent headache pattern, but it
may be intermittent initially.

IV. Subacute, Persistent, Progressive Headache
A. Description

This category frequently includes those illnesses that have
a subacute onset and a progressive course, although inter-

mittent pain may be present initially. Table 4.7 lists the key conditions characterized by subacute, persistent, and progressive headache patterns.

B. Selected Topics
1. Chronic subdural hematoma

Chronic subdural hematoma can produce severe or milder forms of progressive, bilateral or unilateral headache, at times with an insidious onset and fluctuating intensity. Changes in cognition, personality, and neurological signs are common accompaniments. Less than half of the patients give a prior history of head trauma. Thus, a high index of suspicion is necessary to make the diagnosis. Cranial percussion tenderness may occur over the site of hematoma.

2. Brain tumor

Headache occurs as the presenting symptom of *brain tumor* in approximately 40% of patients. The headache is usually generalized but can overlie the tumor. The headaches may be mild to moderate in severity, and commonly are accompanied by nausea and vomiting (seen in about one-half of patients). If an intermittent and throbbing pattern is present, differentiation from migraine is difficult. Altered position, coughing, or exertion may aggravate the headache in approximately 25% of patients. Morning awakening with headache is common. A progressive pattern eventually occurs. Brain tumors may undergo spontaneous, parenchymal hemorrhage.

TABLE 4.7. **CONDITIONS ASSOCIATED WITH SUBACUTE, PERSISTENT, PROGRESSIVE HEADACHE**

Chronic subdural hematoma
Brain tumor
Brain abscess
Cerebral vein thrombosis, including cavernous sinus thrombosis
Idiopathic intracranial hypertension (pseudotumor cerebri)
Central nervous system (CNS) infection (fungal, Lyme, viral meningitis, etc.)
Temporal and cerebral arteritis
Migraine and its variants
Hemicrania continua
Progressive metabolic abnormalities (hypoxia, renal or liver failure, hypercapnia, etc.)
Headache associated with substances or their withdrawal
Cerebrospinal fluid (CSF) hypotension
Cervical spine, occipitocervical junction disease
Dental, cranial vault, temporomandibular (TM) joint disease
Cranial, paranasal sinusitis (see Chapter 11; see Druce, 1991)

3. Brain abscess

The headache of *brain abscess* is similar to that of brain tumor. However, the course is usually more rapid. Associated meningitis and/or other signs of infection may be evident.

4. Idiopathic, benign, intracranial hypertension (pseudotumor cerebri)

Pseudotumor cerebri, also called *idiopathic* or *benign intracranial hypertension*, is associated with headache that appears to correlate with pressure elevation, but which may have features more reminiscent of migraine variants including daily, persistent headache. Visual obscuration and papilledema are noted in most but not all cases. The condition is most common in obese women, often with hormonal or endocrine disturbances. It has been reported following administration of antibiotics and danocrine, as well as other agents. Diagnosis must be established by lumbar puncture that demonstrates elevation of cerebral spinal fluid pressure.

Headaches characteristically, but not always, improve following a lumbar puncture. *Approximately 5–10% of patients do not demonstrate papilledema, particularly in chronic cases, due to changes in the optic disc.* (See Chapter 16 for a more complete discussion.)

5. Giant cell arteritis (temporal arteritis)

Temporal arteritis is a painful inflammation of the cranial arteries, associated with systemic signs and symptoms, including general malaise, myalgias, arthralgias, and anemia. Headache, the most consistent complaint, may localize anywhere about the scalp but is most often in the temples (half of cases). The condition often begins insidiously and may persist for weeks, months, or years. Jaw claudication, orbital pain, anorexia, weight loss, and diaphoresis may be accompaniments.

Sudden visual loss or stroke-like symptoms are the most serious complications of temporal arteritis. The diagnosis is made by clinical history, the presence of a tender, nonpulsatile artery, and an elevation of erythrocyte sedimentation rate (range 60–120 mm Westergren). *A normal or only modestly elevated sedimentation rate is seen in 25% of patients.* Temporal artery biopsy and/or arteriography are generally required to confirm the diagnosis.

Most cases of temporal arteritis occur in persons after the age of 50, but the condition has been reported in younger patients.

Steroid therapy is the treatment of choice.

6. CSF infection

Benign viral meningitis may present with subacute severe headache associated with mild nuchal rigidity and significant photophobia. The CSF usually demonstrates the presence of mild to moderate leukocytosis. The condition is generally self-limited, but the headache requires treatment. Short-term analgesic administration seems most appropriate.

Systemic viruses may either spread directly to the CNS or impart "remote effects," in which direct spread is not apparent. Persistent headache, mood and mental disturbances, sleep abnormalities, and fatigue, among other phenomena, are common. Current speculation suggests that neurotransmitter/receptor disturbances result from either direct viral involvement or remote influence on CNS mechanisms. The *chronic fatigue syndrome* may be the most apparent example.

Acquired immune deficiency syndrome (AIDS) is a disturbance of cell-mediated immunity resulting in opportunistic infections and demyelinating disorders. Headache may be the presenting symptom in persons with CNS involvement and is most likely caused by cryptococcal meningitis and other HIV-related meningitides. The headache is generalized and diffuse and is most prominent in the frontal and occipital regions. Nausea and vomiting are common.

MRI and lumbar puncture are key diagnostic interventions.

(For other meningitides or encephalitis, including those caused by herpes simplex, Lyme disease, and others, consult standard neurological textbooks.)

7. Sinusitis

The role of sinusitis as a cause or aggravating influence for headache is controversial. Most authorities would agree that *acute sinusitis*, and probably *subacute sinusitis* as well, cause headache or contribute to existing pain syndromes. The role of chronic sinusitis is more controversial, and many contend that it too can contribute a headache-producing influence. An excellent review of sinusitis, with guidelines and recommendations for the evaluation, can be found in the reference Druce, 1991. When present, aggressive treatment is indicated. Surgical intervention is strongly discouraged, except in extreme circumstances and when conservative treatment fails, since it is likely to make matters worse if performed primarily to control intractable headache.

Summary

The clinician must have a broad perspective when considering the differential diagnosis of headache. The overlapping that is apparent in the various presentations listed in this chapter reflects the difficulty in approaching this challenge within the limits of any one strategy.

5

Medications Used in the Pharmacotherapy of Headache

Introduction

This chapter contains a comprehensive review of the pharmacological agents used to treat various types of head, face, and neck pain. Also included are numerous tables, charts, and other listings to provide the reader with a detailed reference (Tables 5.22 and 5.23). At the end of this book are additional tables that might be useful.

This chapter should be used in conjunction with subsequent chapters in which treatment recommendations are provided for specific clinical entities.

Special Warning

Many of the agents recommended in this chapter for the treatment of headache and pain have not been approved for such usage by the FDA. Moreover, many of the drugs that are listed, while widely administered, have not been subjected to well-controlled studies to determine efficacy. The reader is cautioned to take these considerations into account when selecting medications.

Also, as mentioned in the Preface, various listings in this chapter will contain the word "selected." Its use designates that an arbitrary choice of items was made, based upon the authors' judgement. Particularly in the case of side effects and contraindications, the reader must take full responsibility to obtain complete and comprehensive prescribing and safety information. This book is intended to serve as a guide only.

Finally, many of the drugs noted in this chapter are not recommended for standard treatment. Their inclusion is to inform the reader as to available treatments for resistant, severe cases. Many of these agents should be administered only by experienced physicians with advanced knowledge of headache and prescribing information about these agents. Moreover, many of these drugs should be given only to resistant cases of severe headache, in settings where careful monitoring and frequent visits, patient education, and safety procedures can be provided. Before administering any of the medications recommended in this text, the physician must consider the clinical circumstances individually and carefully. Keep in mind that pharmacotherapeutic needs vary widely between patients. Also, while every effort was made to ensure accuracy in this book, printing errors may have occurred. It is always best to verify dosages.

I. Symptomatic Treatment vs. Preventive Treatment

A. Symptomatic (Abortive) Treatment

The *symptomatic treatment* of head pain involves the use of agents that reverse, abort, or reduce pain once it has begun or is anticipated.

Generally (exceptions exist), the use of symptomatic medication should not exceed two, and at the most three, days per week. Symptomatic treatment *alone* should be considered when:

- Attacks are infrequent (two or less per week);
- Preventive medication is contraindicated; and
- Compliance to preventive medicine regimens is not achievable.

For frequent attacks, a combination of preventive and symptomatic treatment is often necessary.

The route of administration can be critical. Gastric emptying delay (gastroparesis) is common during acute attacks of migraine and related headaches. Rectal or parenteral forms of medication are of particular value in such instances. Lessening or reversal of gastroparesis can be achieved by pretreatment with metoclopramide.

B. Preventive Treatment

Preventive (prophylactic) treatment is used to prevent attacks and reduce the frequency and severity of headache events. It is appropriate when:

- Attacks of acute pain occur more than two times per week;
- The severity or duration of attacks justifies the use of preventive treatment, even if attacks occur less often than twice per week;
- Symptomatic medication is not effective for infrequent attacks;
- Symptomatic treatment cannot be used because of medical contraindication; and
- To enhance the efficacy of symptomatic medication.

In most instances in which preventive treatment is employed, symptomatic medication must also be used for the treatment of acute attacks that escape preventive measures.

II. Drugs Used to Treat Headache and Face Pain: Symptomatic

(*Note to readers*: At the end of this chapter and the book are various tables and summaries that might be of additional value when considering drug treatment of head and face pain.)

A. Analgesics and Analgesic Combinations (see Table 5.1)

1. General comments

Analgesics are appropriate for the treatment of infrequent, mild to moderate headache, or very severe headaches unresponsive to more specific treatment. Drugs in this group include simple analgesics, such as aspirin and acetaminophen, combination analgesics, and narcotics.

Though generally safe when used infrequently, a major disadvantage of this group of drugs is the potential for overuse.

Advocates of combination analgesics justify their use with the following points:

- Enhanced analgesia from multiple mechanisms of action;
- Enhancement of GI absorption (caffeine); and
- Enhanced control of anxiety via tranquilization; a primary effect on the pain mechanism from barbiturates.

2. Proposed mechanisms

a. Aspirin—prostaglandin synthesis inhibitor
b. Acetaminophen—prostaglandin synthesis inhibitor within the central nervous system; a proposed effect on endorphin/opiate system
c. Narcotics—stimulation of endogenous opiate receptors
d. Caffeine—stimulation of adenosine receptors; enhanced analgesia; increased GI absorption

3. Recommended use

The aforementioned treatments may be used in all infrequently occurring head and face pain disorders. *Children should avoid aspirin for headache, since the headache event may be an early component of a viral syndrome that serves as a prelude to Reye's syndrome.*

4. Principles of use (see Table 5.21)

In general, analgesics should not be used more than two days per week, and more ideally less often, due to "*rebound phenomenon.*" (See Chapters 7–9). More frequent use may be justified during self-limited and defined episodes of pain, such as menstrual periods. It may also be acceptable in limited numbers of patients in whom frequent use of analgesics, including opiates, is considered justifiable because of health or intractable pain considerations (see below).

5. Drugs in this group (see Table 5.1)

Many other oral and parenteral agents, including agonist/antagonist agents, are available. See Table 5.2 for the caffeine content of analgesic preparations and foods. See Table 5.3 for opiate equivalency estimates.

The use of opiates in the treatment of benign head pain is controversial. However, many authorities believe that clinical circumstances exist in which the use of opiates is justified. Frequent use of opiates can be considered in patients without a past profile of overusage or dependency/ addiction, who have severe, debilitating pain and cannot take other medications safely or effectively.

TABLE 5.1. **SELECTED ANALGESIC PREPARATIONS**

Simple analgesics and analgesic combinations	
Aspirin	
Tylenol	
Mixed over-the-counter preparations	
Combination analgesics containing barbiturates	
Fiorinal	aspirin 325 mg, caffeine 40 mg, butalbital 50 mg
Fioricet, Esgic	acetaminophen 325 mg, caffeine 40 mg, butalbital 50 mg
Phrenilin	acetaminophen 325 mg, butalbital 50 mg
Combination analgesics containing codeine	
Fiorinal w/codeine	aspirin 325 mg, caffeine 40 mg, butalbital 50 mg, codeine 30 mg
Tylenol w/codeine III	acetaminophen 325 mg, codeine 30 mg
Phrenilin w/codeine	acetaminophen 325 mg, butalbital 50 mg, codeine 30 mg
Narcotic analgesics/analgesics containing narcotics	
Darvon CPD-65	propoxyphene HCL 65 mg, aspirin 389 mg, caffeine 32.4 mg
Darvocet-N	propoxyphene napsylate 50/100 mg, acetaminophen 325 mg
Vicodin	hydrocodone 5 mg, acetaminophen 500 mg
Percocet	oxycodone 5 mg, acetaminophen 325 mg
Percodan	oxycodone 4.5 mg, aspirin 325 mg
Demerol	meperidine 50/100 mg tablet; injectable
Dilaudid	hydromorphone 1/2/3/4 mg tablets 3 mg suppository 2 mg/ml injections
Stadol	butorphanol (IV, IM, or nasal spray)

TABLE 5.2. **CAFFEINE CONTENT OF COMMON FOODS AND DRUGS**

Product	Example	Caffeine Content (mg)
Cocoa and chocolate	Baking chocolate (1 oz)	35
	Chocolate candy bar	25
	Cocoa beverage (6 oz mixture)	10
	Milk chocolate (1 oz)	6
Coffee	Decaffeinated (5 oz)	2
	Drip (5 oz)	146
	Instant, regular (5 oz)	53
	Percolated (5 oz)	110
Over-the-counter drugs	Anacin	32
	Excedrin	65
	No-Doz tablets	100–200
	Vanquish	33
	Vivarin tablets	200
Prescription drugs	Darvon	32.4
	Esgic	40
	Fioricet	40
	Fiorinal	40
	Norgesic	30
	Norgesic Forte	60
	Supac	33
	Synalgos-DC	30
Soft drinks (12 oz)	7-Up/Diet 7-Up	0
	Coca-Cola	34
	Diet Pepsi	34
	Dr. Pepper	38
	Fresca	0
	Ginger Ale	0
	Hires Root Beer	0
	Mountain Dew	52
	Pepsi-Cola	37
	Tab	44
Tea	1-minute brew (5 oz)	9–33
	3-minute brew (5 oz)	22–46
	5-minute brew (5 oz)	20–50
	Canned ice tea (12 oz)	22–36

Opiates may provide effective pain control in those who would otherwise not achieve it. Moreover, there is growing sentiment that physicians have the obligation to provide effective pain relief when possible. The risks of opiate therapy are at times minimal compared with the impact upon patient, family, and society when severe pain is not effectively treated or when large (toxic) amounts of more "acceptable" agents are required.

TABLE 5.3. **SELECTED OPIATE (OR ANTAGONIST/AGONIST) EQUIVALENCY ESTIMATES COMPARED WITH 10 MG INTRAMUSCULAR MORPHINE SULFATE**[a]

Drug	Trade Name	Equivalent Parenteral Dose (mg)	Equivalent PO Dose (mg)
Anileridine	Leritine	25	75
Buprenorphine[b]	Buprenex	0.3	—
Butorphanol[b]	Stadol	2.0	
Codeine phosphate	Codeine	120	200
Diphenoxylate	Lomotil	—	300
Fentanyl	Sublimaze/Innovar	0.1	—
Hydrocodone	Hycodan, Vicodin	—	10–15
Hydromorphone	Dilaudid	2	4
Levorphanol tartrate	Levo-Dromoran	2	4
Meperidine	Demerol	75	300
Methadone	Dolophine	10	20
Morphine		10	20–30
Immediate-release	Roxanol	10	20–60
Controlled-release	Roxanol SR	—	20–60
Nalbuphine[b]	Nubain	10–15	—
Naloxone[c]	Narcan		
Naltrexone[c]	Trexan		
Oxycodone w/ASA	Percodan	—	10–15
Oxycodone w/ACET	Percocet	—	10–15
Oxymorphone	Numorphan	1	—
Pentazocine[b]	Talwin	60	180
Propoxyphene	Darvon	—	120

[a]Modified from the Analgesic Study Section, Sloan-Kettering Institute for Cancer Research, New York, and Purdue Frederick, Inc., Toronto.
[b]Agonist/antagonist.
[c]Pure antagonist.

6. Selected major untoward reactions and contraindications

    a. Aspirin—asthma, rash, gastrointestinal irritation, effects on coagulation

    b. Acetaminophen—liver toxicity and high dose may potentiate oral anticoagulants; chronic use may contribute to renal disturbances

    c. Narcotics—nausea, vomiting, respiratory depression, sedation, constipation, addiction and/or dependence

    d. Barbiturates—drowsiness, addiction, effects on coagulation

    All drugs in this group can potentially produce "rebounding" when used frequently. Low-dose aspirin may be an exception.

    See standard references for additional untoward reactions, guidelines, contraindications, and warnings.

B. Nonsteroidal Anti-Inflammatory Drugs
1. General comments

Numerous nonsteroidal anti-inflammatory drugs (NSAIDs) are available. Though similar in many ways, the analgesic effect may differ between agents. They are potentially useful in both symptomatic and preventive regimens, but it is advisable to avoid prolonged, frequent use for safety reasons.

2. Proposed mechanisms

The proposed mechanisms of agents in this group include:

a. Inhibition of cyclooxygenase (inhibits prostaglandin synthesis)
b. Inhibition of lipooxygenase (inhibits leukotriene synthesis)
c. Prostaglandin receptor antagonism
d. Interference with cell-membrane processes

3. Recommended use

a. Mild to moderate migraine and tension-type headache
b. Exertional and menstrual headache
c. Benign orgasmic cephalgia
d. Chronic paroxysmal hemicrania (indomethacin)
e. Hemicrania continua (indomethacin)
f. "Icepick" syndromes (indomethacin)
g. Acute or intractable migraine (parenteral ketorolac)

4. Principles of use (see Table 5.21)

These agents should be taken at the first sign of a headache or for reliably anticipated attacks. Ordinarily, administration should not exceed three usage days per week, but more frequent, continuous use for defined, self-limited periods of time may be acceptable, such as around a menstrual period.

5. Selected drugs in this group (see Table 5.4)
6. Selected major untoward reactions and contraindications

a. Major untoward reactions
1) GI ulcers/bleeding
2) Oral ulcers
3) Colitis activation/aggravation
4) Headache, lightheadedness, and dizziness
5) Somnolence
6) Tinnitus

TABLE 5.4. **SELECTED NONSTEROIDAL ANTI-INFLAMMATORY DRUGS**

Type	Available Size (mg)
Carboxylic acids	
Acetylated	
Aspirin	
Nonacetylated	
Choline magnesium	
trisalicylate (Trilisate)	500/750/1000
Salsalate (Salflex, Disalcid)	500/750
Propionic acids	
Ibuprofen (Motrin, Advil)	200/400/600
Naproxen (Naprosyn)	250/375/500
Fenoprofen (Nalfon)	200/300/600
Naproxen sodium (Anaprox)	275/550
Ketoprofen (Orudis)	25/50/75
Aryl and heterocyclic acids	
Tolmetin (Tolectin)	200/400/600
Indomethacin (Indocin)	25/50/75
	50 rectal
Diclofenac (Voltaren)	25/50/75
Sulindac (Clinoril)	150/200
Fenamic acids	
Mefenamic acid (Ponstel)	250
Meclofenamate (Meclomen)	50/100
Enolic acids	
Phenylbutazone (Butazolidine)	100
Piroxicam (Feldene)	10/20
Pyrrolo-pyrrole	
Ketorolac (Toradol) (IM)	15/30/60
Ketorolac (Toradol) (PO)	10

    7) Fluid retention

    8) Asthma activation/aggravation

    9) Hypertension aggravation

  b. Contraindications/cautionary recommendations

    1) Active ulcer disease

    2) Gastritis

    3) Renal disease

    4) Bleeding disorders

    5) Aspirin-sensitive asthma

    6) Severe hypertension

    7) Colitis (active or in remission—a relative contraindication)

     See standard references for additional untoward reactions, guidelines, contraindications, and warnings.

7. Special considerations

    Recently, parenteral ketorolac has become available for treatment of acute headache syndromes. The preliminary impression is that it has value as a parenteral, symptomatic therapy.

Frequent use of NSAIDs requires monitoring of GI blood loss, renal function, and blood pressure. The therapeutic dose may vary from patient to patient. If failure to respond to one agent occurs, another should be tried.

C. Ergotamine Derivatives
1. General comments

Ergotamine derivatives remain the drugs of first choice for moderate to severe migraine and related headaches. They are available for headache in the form of ergotamine tartrate (Cafergot, etc.), as well as dihydroergotamine (DHE). Ergot alkaloids are derived from the rye fungus (Claviceps purpurea) (see Table 5.5).

DHE is an ergot derivative that has been reduced at the 9–10 double bond on the D-lysergic acid moiety. It differs from ergotamine tartrate in the following important ways:

- It is a *weak* arterial vasoconstrictor (ergotamine tartrate is a more potent arterial constrictor);
- It has selective venoconstricting properties;
- It has substantially less emetic (nauseating) properties; and
- It has less uterine effects.

2. Proposed mechanisms

Both ergotamine tartrate and DHE have:
a. Agonist actions on 5-HT_{1a} and 5-HT_{1d}, as well as α-adrenergic receptors
b. Vasoconstriction effects via stimulation of arterial smooth muscle through 5-HT receptors
c. Venous capacitance vessel constriction
d. Reuptake inhibition of noradrenalin at sympathetic nerve endings
e. Reduction of vasogenic/neurogenic inflammation

A fundamental action of ergot derivatives on migraine may be via inhibition of neurogenic inflammation of the trigeminal vascular system, not via vasoconstriction. Central neurotransmitter effects are also likely. DHE passes through the blood-brain barrier and localizes to nuclei in the brainstem and spinal cord involved in pain transmission and modulation.

3. Recommended use

Ergot derivatives are appropriate in the symptomatic treatment of the following conditions:

    a. Moderate to severe migraine (DHE, ergotamine tartrate)

    b. Cluster headache

    c. Intractable migraine (status migrainosis) (DHE)

    d. Intractable, chronic daily headache (DHE)

4. Principles of use (see Table 5.21)

    a. Ergotamine tartrate—ergotamine tartrate is appropriate for acute attacks of migraine. For accompanying or induced nausea, treatment with antinauseants is recommended. Because of concern for "rebound" and ergot dependency syndrome (see later and Table 5.8), it is advisable to limit its use to 2 days per week, except perhaps for cluster headache or menstrual migraine, during which more extended but still limited usage is acceptable.

    b. DHE—DHE is given intravenously (IV), intramuscularly (IM), or subcutaneously (SC) and is appropriate for:

       • Acute, individual attacks of migraine or cluster headache

       • Prolonged intractable attacks

For prolonged intractable attacks, DHE should be used in a 3–5 day intravenous protocol (see Table 5.6, Fig. 5.1, and Chapter 6).

DHE is also very effective in treating cluster headache and menstrual migraine and controlling headache during rebound and detoxification of patients who have excessively used ergotamine tartrate or analgesics for frequent headaches. Self-injected subcutaneous DHE is appropriate for reliable patients with occasional, severe headache. DHE is relatively unstable and poorly soluble in other solutions. It is best administered immediately after removing it from the ampule.

TABLE 5.5. **SELECTED SYMPTOMATIC DRUGS CONTAINING ERGOT DERIVATIVES**

Cafergot suppositories/tablets
Wigraine suppositories/tablets
Ergomar sublingual tablets
Ergostat sublingual tablets
Migrogot tablets
DHE–45

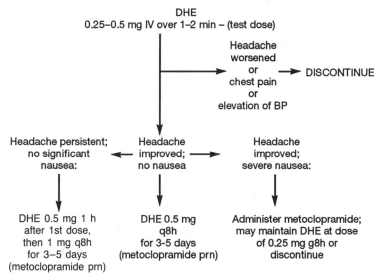

Figure 5.1 IV DHE Administration Algorithm.

TABLE 5.6. **INTRAVENOUS PROTOCOL FOR DIHYDROERGOTAMINE (DHE) ADMINISTRATION**

Protocol
- 0.25–0.5 mg IV "push" (test dose), over 2 minutes via heparin lock apparatus.
- If tolerated, DHE 0.5–1 mg IV "push" q 8 hours for 3–5 days.
- Administer 10 mg metoclopramide (IV[a] or IM) before DHE administration, if nausea occurs.
- Maintain for 3–5 days, if tolerated. May repeat program one time.

Guidelines for use
1. Administer metoclopramide before or at DHE administration if necessary to control nausea. Discontinue if not necessary.
2. DHE to be administered via 1–2 minute slow "push."
3. Most patients stabilize at end of day 3, but extension of program for 2–3 more days may be necessary.
4. Discontinue DHE via a 1–3 day gradual reduction program if patient is pain-free for 2 days or fails to respond after 3 days.
5. Hospitalization is most appropriate for therapy, during which careful monitoring for blood pressure elevation, chest pain, severe nausea, etc. can be carried out and necessary concurrent therapies can be administered, including establishment of an effective preventive program.
6. Discontinue or substantially reduce dose if severe nausea, chest pain, severe leg cramps, or other significant adverse reactions occur.

[a]10 mg slow "IV push" or in 50 cc 5% dextrose in water (D5W) over 20–30 minutes.

5. Selected drugs in this group (see Table 5.5)
6. Selected major untoward reactions and contraindications

All ergotamine preparations are capable of producing nausea, vomiting, paresthesias, muscle cramps, and angina in sensitive individuals. Initially, low-dose administration may be helpful in reducing symptoms. Continued usage at symptom-producing doses should be avoided. These effects are generally less likely with DHE.

For contraindications and cautionary warnings, see Table 5.7.

7. Special considerations

Frequent use of ergotamine tartrate—more than two days per week—can result in ergot dependency (see Table 5.8) This condition will be discussed further in Chapters 6, 7, and 9.

TABLE 5.7. **CONTRAINDICATIONS TO ERGOT DERIVATIVES**[a]

Age over 60 years (relative contraindication)
Pregnancy
Breast-feeding
Bradycardia (moderate to severe)
Cardiac valvular disease (moderate to severe)
Collagen vascular disease, vasculitis
Coronary artery disease
Hypertension (moderate to severe)
Impaired hepatic or renal function (moderate to severe)
Infection or fever/sepsis (enhances vasoconstriction)
Peptic ulcer disease
Peripheral vascular disease
Cerebral vascular disease
Severe pruritus

[a]See standard references for additional untoward reactions, guidelines, contraindications, and warnings. Avoid ergot-containing agents in pregnancy, and encourage effective birth control methods in patients using these medications.

TABLE 5.8. **SYNDROME OF ERGOTAMINE TARTRATE DEPENDENCE**[a]

Ergotamine tartrate dependence is characterized by:
1. The initial presence of intermittent migraine;
2. Insidious increase of headache frequency and ergotamine tartrate usage;
3. The dependable and irresistible use of ergotamine tartrate as the only effective agent; and
4. Attempts to discontinue the medication results in intensification of pain and accompaniments (withdrawal), thereby promoting continual usage.

[a]"Rebounding" is not currently believed to occur with dihydroergotamine usage, but the question remains open.

Table 5.9 provides a listing of the components of selected ergotamine preparations. Table 5.10 provides a mechanism for determining the subnauseating dose of the ergot preparations.

Bioavailability of ergotamine tartrate is dependent upon route of administration. Oral absorption is erratic, but rectal absorption provides a substantial increase and is generally considered 85–90% effective when taken appropriately for acute migraine.

Pretreatment with antiemetic agents is advisable when nausea occurs as part of the migraine or is induced by the ergot derivative and cannot be avoided at therapeutic doses (see page 51 and Table 5.21).

D. Isometheptene

1. General comments

The most well-known agent containing isometheptene is Midrin. Midrin is a combination of three active ingredients: isometheptene mucate, 65 mg; acetaminophen, 325 mg; dichloralphenazone 100 mg. The combination is effective for symptomatic treatment of mild to moderate migraine and migraine-like headaches and is usually quite safe and well tolerated. The combination is of particular value in patients who cannot take ergotamine tartrate but require an orally administered antimigraine drug.

TABLE 5.9. **COMPONENTS OF SELECTED ERGOT DERIVATIVES**

Cafergot (oral tablet)	ergotamine tartrate 1 mg, caffeine 100 mg
Wigraine (oral tablet)	ergotamine tartrate 1 mg, caffeine 100 mg
Cafergot (rectal suppository)	ergotamine tartrate 2 mg, caffeine 100 mg
Ergostat (sublingual)	ergotamine tartrate 2 mg
Ergomar (sublingual)	ergotamine tartrate 2 mg
Dihydroergotamine	dihydroergotamine 1 mg/ml ampules (IM, SC, IV)

TABLE 5.10. **PREDETERMINING SUBNAUSEATING DOSE OF ERGOT DERIVATIVES (OPTIONAL)**[a]

1. Advise patient to start with one tablet, or 1/4 suppository, or 1/2 sublingual tablet of ergotamine tartrate when not experiencing a headache. Experiment with increasing dose in separate trials until nausea occurs.
2. Determine the highest subnauseating dose.
3. Select the appropriate form and dose.

[a]The need to establish a subnauseating dose is variable and optional. It is often not necessary, but for patients who are frightened of the nausea or are severely affected, predetermination may be advisable.

2. Proposed mechanisms

The mechanism of action reflects individual components. Isometheptene mucate is a sympathomimetic vaso-active agent, which probably impacts headaches centrally. Acetaminophen has analgesic properties, and dichloral-phenazone, a tranquilizing agent, may affect central pain mechanisms.

3. Recommended use

a. Mild to moderate migraine
b. Tension-type headache (probably a migraine variant)

4. Principles of use (see Table 5.21)

Isometheptene compounds should be used for symptomatic treatment and can be combined with nonsteroidal anti-inflammatory agents for greater efficacy. Short-term, self-limited, daily use around menstrual periods or for prolonged migraine is generally acceptable.

5. Drugs in this group

Midrin
Isocom

6. Selected major untoward reactions and contraindications

Drugs containing isometheptene are contraindicated in patients using monoamine oxidase inhibitors (MAO) inhibitors and patients with partial spinal cord lesions due to sympathomimetic stimulation and severe hypertensive reactions.

a. Common untoward reactions:
  • Transient dizziness
  • Sedation
b. Contraindications/cautionary warnings:
  1) Glaucoma
  2) Severe renal disease
  3) Severe hypertension
  4) Severe heart or liver disease
  5) MAOI therapy
  6) In patients with spinal cord lesions

See standard references for additional untoward reactions, guidelines, contraindications, and warnings.

E. Corticosteroids

1. General comments

Corticosteroids have long been considered effective in the treatment of many headache conditions but are most appropriate for cluster headache and prolonged, intractable attacks of migraine. In addition to the well-known risks of corticosteroid therapy, more recently, concern has increased regarding the possible development of avascular necrosis, particularly, but not exclusively, of the hip. Though extremely rare when considering the frequency with which steroids are administered, the condition has been reported with both occasional, low-dose and prolonged, high-dose usage. Proper informed consent is advisable.

2. Proposed mechanisms

The mechanism by which steroids affect headache remains uncertain. The following are possible:

   a. Anti-inflammatory effect on neurogenic inflammation

   b. Reduction of vasogenic edema

   c. Effects on central aminergic/serotonergic mechanisms

3. Recommended use

   a. Cluster headache
   - When refractory to other agents
   - For breakthrough attacks
   - At onset of treatment to provide immediate control

   b. Intractable migraine

   c. Altitudinal headache

   d. Headaches associated with increased intracranial pressure/edema

For cluster headache or intractable migraine, a short-term "tapering" course of oral steroids is recommended (see Table 5.11).

4. Principles of use (see Table 5.21)

Steroids should be used according to general prescribing guidelines and restrictions. For intractable, severe headaches (migraine, cluster headache), intravenous regimens are available (see Chapter 6). Steroid treatment is best reserved for circumstances in which other appropriate agents have failed or are contraindicated and in patients with severe, acute, protracted conditions.

5. Selected drugs in this group (see Tables 5.12 and 5.13)

6. Selected major untoward reactions and contraindications

   a. Osteoporosis (with prolonged use)

   b. Diabetes (aggravation)

   c. Hypertension (aggravation)

TABLE 5.11. **RECOMMENDED PREDNISONE PROGRAM FOR 7- AND 10-DAY TREATMENT**[a]

	7-Day Prednisone Program (5 mg tablets—dispense 60 tablets)		
Day	Breakfast (mg)	Lunch (mg)	Dinner (mg)
1	20 (4 pills)	20	20
2	20	20	20
3	20	15 (3 pills)	15
4	15	15	10 (2 pills)
5	10	10	10
6	10	5 (1 pill)	5
7	5	5	

	10-Day Prednisone Program (5 mg tablets—dispense 80 tablets)		
Day	Breakfast (mg)	Lunch (mg)	Dinner (mg)
1	20 (4 pills)	20	20
2	20	20	20
3	20	20	20
4	20	20	20
5	20	15 (3 pills)	15
6	15	15	10 (2 pills)
7	10	10	10
8	10	5 (1 pill)	5
9	5		5
10	5		

[a]Predisone should not be used if infection, an ulcer, or pregnancy is present. (Consult standard references for contraindications.) Aspirin and other nonsteroidal anti-inflammatory drugs should be avoided while taking prednisone.
WARNING: Steroid use has been associated in rare instances with avascular necrosis.

TABLE 5.12. **SELECTED STEROIDS AND DOSE**

Prednisone	PO 40–100 mg per day, then taper. Avoid prolonged or repetitive use, if possible
Dexamethasone (Decadron)	PO, IM, or IV 8–20 mg per day. Avoid prolonged or repetitive use, if possible
Hydrocortisone	IV 100–500 mg per day. See Chapter 6. Avoid prolonged or repetitive use, if possible
Methylprednisolone (Solu-Medrol)	IV 100–500 mg per day. Avoid prolonged or repetitive use, if possible

TABLE 5.13. **COMPARISON OF SELECTED CORTICOSTEROID DRUG PROFILES**[a]

Drug	Potency	Na⁺ Retention[a]	Duration of Action[b]	Equivalent Dose (mg)[e]
6-α-methyl-prednisolone	5	0.5	I	4
β-methasone	25	0	L	0.75
Corticosterone	0.35	15	S	—
Cortisol (hydrocortisone)	1	1	S	20
Cortisone (11-Dehydrocortisol)	0.8	0.8	S	25
Dexamethasone	25	0	L	0.75
Paramethasone	10	0	L	2
Prednisolone	4	0.8	I	5
Prednisone	4	0.8	I	5
Triamcinolone	5	0	I	4

[a]Modified and abstracted from Timothy Covington, Pharm. D. et al. Drug facts and comparisons, 1989 ed. The pharmalogical basis of therapeutics. 8th ed. J. B. Lippincott & Co. St. Louis, MO, p. 1447.
[b]Relative anti-inflammatory potency.
[c]Relative mineralocorticoid (sodium-retaining) potency.
[d]Duration of action: S = Short-acting (8–12 hrs)
                        I = Intermediate-acting (18–36 hrs)
                        L = Long-acting (36–54 hrs)
[e]Approximate equivalent dose (mg), as applied to oral or intravenous administration

    d. Myopathy
    e. Avascular necrosis of femoral and humeral head (rare but increasingly reported)
    f. Steroid dependence and Cushing's syndrome
    See standard references for additional untoward reactions, guidelines, contraindications, and warnings.

F. Phenothiazines/Neuroleptics

1. General comments

Phenothiazines and other neuroleptics are generally used for symptomatic relief of pain and for the treatment of nausea and vomiting. Phenothiazines are available in oral, rectal, and parenteral forms.

2. Proposed mechanisms

The phenothiazine/neuroleptic effect on headache and nausea is via an influence on 5–HT₃ receptors and dopamine receptors (antagonist). Metoclopramide also enhances gastric motility.

3. Recommended use

    a. Control of nausea/vomiting
    b. Symptomatic therapy of migraine and cluster headache

4. Principles of use (see Table 5.21)

Drugs in this group should be given by rectal or parenteral route for nausea and vomiting. They also may be useful for symptomatic treatment of pain by oral, rectal, or parenteral route.

See Chapter 6 for intravenous protocol using chlorpromazine or prochlorperazine.

5. **Selected drugs in this group**
   a. chlorpromazine (Thorazine)
   b. prochlorperazine (Compazine)
   c. perphenazine (Trilafon)
   d. pimozide (Orap)—recently recommended for facial neuralgia
   e. metoclopramide (Reglan)
   f. promethazine (Phenergan)
   g. trimethobenzamide (Tigan)

6. **Selected major untoward reactions and contraindications**
   a. **Common untoward reactions of phenothiazine and neuroleptic agents**
      1) Extrapyramidal reactions (acute dystonia, tardive dyskinesia, akathisia, Parkinsonism, etc.)
      2) Hypotension (particularly with parenteral usage)
      3) Sedation/confusion
      4) Anticholinergic effects
   b. **Contraindications/cautionary warnings:**
      1) Severe hypotension
      2) Particular vulnerability to extrapyramidal reactions
      3) Previous adverse reactions
      4) Conditions worsened by anticholinergic effects
         • narrow-angle glaucoma
         • prostatism
         • some cardiac arrythmias
         • others

   See standard references for additional untoward reactions, guidelines, contraindications, and warnings.

7. **Special considerations**

   Extrapyramidal reactions (dystonia, akathisia) may respond to diphenhydramine (Benadryl, 25–50 mg), via oral, intramuscular, or intravenous route.

   While useful for acute headache treatment, and even prevention in some instances, phenothiazine and related medications should be restricted to symptomatic treatment of nausea/vomiting, except in selected instances when severe pain is refractory to more standard treatment.

G. Sumatriptan (Imitrex)

1. General comments

At the time of this writing, sumatriptan has not yet been approved for the U.S. market, and therefore the description of this drug will be limited. Sumatriptan is a selective $5-HT_1$ agent and is considered useful for symptomatic treatment of acute migraine and cluster headache.

Sumatriptan is generally considered safe, but side effects are seen in about 62% of patients. These side effects are usually transient and mild. Sumatriptan, like ergot derivatives, has vasoconstrictive properties that may limit its use in cardiac, cerebral, and peripheral vascular disease. Sumatriptan in the oral form is considered effective in decreasing headache to mild or no pain within 2 hours, and subcutaneous administration is 70–73% effective in decreasing headache to mild or no pain. Headache may recur in up to 40% of patients. Sumatriptan may have a particularly beneficial influence in controlling nausea as well as headache.

2. Proposed mechanisms

Sumatriptan is a selective, $5-HT_1$ agonist. It is thought to have its effect in the neurovascular system and, like ergot derivatives, may reverse neurogenic inflammation. There is speculation that it exerts its effect centrally as well.

3. Recommended use

a. Acute, moderate to severe migraine
b. Cluster headache

4. Principles of use

Prescribing details are not available.

5. Drugs in this group

Imitrex

6. Major untoward reactions and contraindications

Must await FDA-approved prescribing information.

III. Drugs Used to Treat Headache and Face Pain: Preventive

The major groups used for the prevention of primary headaches include:

- β-adrenergic blockers;
- Calcium channel antagonists;
- Antidepressants;
- Ergot derivatives (methysergide and related agents);
- Anticonvulsants;

- Nonsteroidal anti-inflammatory agents;
- Lithium (cluster headache); and
- Others (see end of chapter)

All or most preventive agents influence serotonin or serotonin receptor function. Several bind to one or more 5–HT receptor sites and may "downregulate" the receptors. Modulation of serotonergic neurons is also considered a possible effect.

Guidelines for the use of preventive agents include:
- Administer a full course for 1–6 months, if effective;
- Allow at least 1 month usage at therapeutic, tolerable dosage before evaluating effectiveness;
- Use concurrent symptomatic medication carefully and be aware of additive potentially adverse effects (e.g., methysergide when used together with ergotamine tartrate for symptomatic treatment; both are vasoconstrictive); and
- Avoid during pregnancy, and encourage effective birth control.

A. β-Adrenergic Blockers
1. General comments

This is the most widely used group of prophylactic agents for migraine and related headache. In 60–80% of cases they are effective in reducing frequency of headache at least 50%. They are not generally effective in the treatment of cluster headache.

Unlike the other β-adrenergic blockers, nadolol is not metabolized in the liver but excreted principally by the kidneys. This makes nadolol particularly valuable when used in combination with other agents such as tricyclic antidepressants (primarily metabolized in the liver) or in patients who have liver disease.

2. Proposed mechanisms

a. Inhibition of norepinephrine release by blocking prejunctional β-receptors.

b. Delayed reduction in tyrosine hydroxylase activity, which is the rate-limiting step in norepinephrine synthesis.

c. Delayed reduction of locus ceruleus neuron firing rate.

It is generally believed that blocking central β-receptors that interfere with vigilance-enhancing adrenergic pathways is important in headache prevention. Certain β-adrenergic blockers may interact with 5–HT receptors. Cross-modulation of the serotonin system has also been proposed.

Contingent negative variation (CNV) normalizes after β-adrenergic blocking. Migraineurs with elevated CNV scores may respond better to β-adrenergic blocking therapy than those without elevations.

3. Recommended use
a. Migraine
b. Chronic daily headache
c. Other related headache disorders (but not cluster headache)

4. Principles of use (see Table 5.21)

β-adrenergic blocking agents should be initially administered in small, divided dosages, titrating upward to tolerance.

Experience with the sustained action drugs, such as Inderal LA and Corgard, suggests that b.i.d. dosing is superior to once-a-day dosing. Bioavailability of Inderal LA is less than short-acting forms, thus requiring increased total daily dosage.

5. Selected drugs in this group
See Table 5.14.

6. Selected major untoward reactions and contraindications
a. Adverse responses
1) Fatigue
2) Depression and memory disturbances
3) Impotence
4) Reduced tolerance for physical activity
5) Hypotension/bradycardia
6) Weight gain
7) Peripheral vasoconstriction
8) Masking of sympathetic-induced hypoglycemic symptomatology
9) Adverse influence on cholesterol and lipid metabolism
10) Bronchospasm

b. Contraindications/cautionary warnings
1) Congestive heart failure
2) Asthma
3) Significant diabetes/hypoglycemia
4) Bradycardia
5) Hypotension
6) Moderate to severe hyperlipidemia

TABLE 5.14. **SELECTED β-BLOCKER DRUG PROFILES**[a]

Drug	Intrinsic Sympathetic Activity	Lipid Solubility	Oral Bioavail. (%)	Half-Life (hrs) in Plasma
Acebutolol[c] (Sectral)	+	1.9	40	2.6
Atenolol[c] (Tenormin)	0	0.23	50	5–8
Esmolol[c] (Brevibloc)	0	0	0	0.13
Labetalol[b,d] (Normodyne/Trandate)	—	—	20	4–6
Metroprolol[c] (Lopressor)	0	2.15	40	3–4
Nadolol[b] (Corgard)	0	0.7	35	10–20
Pindolol[b] (Visken)	+ +	1.75	75	3–4
Propranolol[b] (Inderal)	0	3.65	25	3–5
Timolol[b] (Blocadren)	0	2.1	50	3–5

0 = nil; + = minimal; + + = minor; + + + = moderate; + + + + = marked.
[a]Modified from Drug Facts and Comparisons. 1989 ed. J. P. Lippincott & Co. St. Louis, MO, p. 234.
[b]Nonselective β (-one and -two) adrenergic antagonist.
[c]Selective β-one adrenergic antagonist.
[d]Labetolol is also a potent α-one adrenergic antagonist.

7) Moderate to severe peripheral vascular disease
8) Vertebrobasilar migraine/complicated migraine
9) Significant cerebrovascular disease
  See standard references for additional untoward reactions, guidelines, contraindications, and warnings.

7. Special considerations

β-blocker therapy must be individualized. If one agent fails, use of another is advisable. *Underdosing is a major cause of therapeutic failure. When discontinuing after extended usage, a gradual reduction program is necessary.*

B. Calcium Channel Antagonists
1. General comments

Calcium channel antagonists (CA) belong to four different chemically heterogenous groups: dihydroproperadines (nifedipine, nimodipine, nicardipine); phenylalkylamines (verapamil); benzothiazepines (diltiazem); and diphenylpiperazines (flunerazine).

Verapamil is the most widely used CA for the treatment of headache. Flunarazine, not available in the U.S., may also have significant efficacy, but adverse effects may limit its usefulness. Nifedipine may produce a worsening of headache in up to 30% of cases.

Verapamil may require several weeks of therapeutic dose administration before beneficial effects are noticeable.

Currently, CAs are not as well established for migraine as are the β-adrenergic blockers, but verapamil is clearly more effective than the β-adrenergic blockers in the treatment of cluster headache.

CAs are more appropriate than β-adrenergic blockers in the treatment of migraine in the following circumstances:

- When bradycardia limits the use of β-adrenergic blockade (calcium antagonists such as verapamil generally do not slow pulse rate significantly);
- In the presence of asthmatic-like conditions;
- In the presence of peripheral or cerebrovascular disease; and
- In the presence of diabetes, hypoglycemia, hyperlipidemia, or complicated migraine

2. Proposed mechanisms

The mechanism of action on headache remains uncertain. The following actions may be important:

a. The ability to block 5–HT release
b. Interference with neurovascular inflammation
c. Interference with initiation and propagation of spreading depression
d. Inhibition of contraction of vascular smooth muscle
e. Inhibition of calcium-dependent enzymes involved in prostaglandin formation
f. Influences on the serotonin systems
g. Prevention of hypoxia on cerebral neurons

3. Recommended use

a. Migraine
b. Cluster headache (verapamil, nimodipine)
c. Daily chronic headache
d. Acute, severe hypertension (sublingual nifedipine)

4. Principles of use (see Table 5.21)

As with β-adrenergic blockers, a small, divided dose should be used initially and then titrated upward to tolerance. High-dose verapamil (160 mg t.i.d. or q.i.d.) appears necessary for beneficial effects in many patients. As with long-acting β-adrenergic blockers, the sustained-release forms of CA have reduced bioavailability, and twice-a-day or even t.i.d. administration may be necessary (beware of excessive dosing.)

5. Drugs in this group
  a. Verapamil (Calan, Isoptin)
  b. Nifedipine (Procardia)
  c. Nimodipine (Nimotop)
  d. Diltiazem (Cardizem)
  e. Flunarazine (Sibelium) (not available in the United States)

6. Selected major untoward reactions and contraindications
  a. **Untoward reactions**
    1) Constipation, A-V block, congestive heart failure, hypotension (verapamil)
    2) Hypotension, reflex tachycardia, headache, nausea and vomiting (nifedipine)
    3) Hypotension, A-V block, headache (diltiazem)
    4) Weight gain, somnolence, dizziness, hypotension, extrapyramidal reactions (flunarazine)
  b. **Contraindications/cautionary warnings:**
    1) Congestive heart failure
    2) Heart block
    3) Moderate to severe bradycardia
    4) Hypotension
    5) Sick sinus syndrome
    6) Atrial flutter or fibrillation
    7) Severe constipation
    See standard references for additional untoward reactions, guidelines, contraindications, and warnings.

C. Antidepressants (TCA)
  See next sections for fluoxetine and MAO inhibitors

1. General comments
  Tricyclic antidepressants (TCAs) are particularly valuable in patients with daily chronic headache, atypical facial pain, and neck pain disorders, with or without depression. They are also effective in many patients with intermittent migraine and related headache forms. Patients with sleep onset difficulties may benefit from sedative TCA given at night.

2. Proposed mechanisms
  a. Increased availability of synaptic norepinephrine or serotonin

b. "Downregulation" of 5–TH$_2$ receptors and decreased β-receptor density
c. Enhancement of opiate mechanisms
d. Inhibition of 5–HT and norepinephrine reuptake

The effect of antidepressants on mood may be related but not fundamental to the effect on headache. When effective for pain, the benefit may occur within days of proper dose administration, whereas depression treatment generally requires several weeks of therapy.

3. Recommended use

a. Migraine and related headaches
b. Episodic and chronic "tension-type" headache, daily chronic headache, etc.
c. Neck pain
d. Facial pain syndromes
e. Pain syndromes accompanied by sleep disturbance or anxiety

4. Principles of use (see Table 5.21)

Generally, TCA should be initially administered as a single dose at bedtime. Exceptions include those drugs which have an activating or stimulating effect, e.g., fluoxetine (not a TCA), desipramine, nortriptyline, and protriptyline. If daytime sedation is present even when a TCA is given at bedtime, switching from a tertiary TCA (amitriptyline, doxepin) to secondary form (nortriptyline, protriptyline) or to fluoxetine may be beneficial. If insomnia or nightmares develop, lowering the dose and/or administering earlier in the day may be helpful.

A therapeutic window may exist below and above which these drugs are ineffective. Thus, individual dosing and monitoring are essential. Moreover, because of the long half-life, drug accumulation is common, and down-dosing is often necessary.

5. Selected drugs in this group

The following drugs are the major TCAs used for headache:

a. Amitriptyline (Elavil, Endep)
b. Nortriptyline (Pamelor, Aventyl)
c. Doxepin (Sinequan, Adapin)
d. Desipramine (Norpramin)
e. Protriptyline (Vivactyl)
f. Others

Other tricyclics and atypical tricyclics are available, such as clomipramine (Anafranil) (see next sections and Table 5.15). The benefit of clomipramine for headache, as with many other TCAs, has yet to be established or has been found to be of relatively little value (as in the case of trazodone—Desyrel).

6. Selected major untoward reactions and contraindications

a. Untoward reactions include:
   1) Weight gain
   2) Dizziness
   3) Tremor/hypomania
   4) Confusion/delirium
   5) May lower seizure threshold
   6) Anticholinergic symptoms, such as
      a) Drowsiness
      b) Dry mouth
      c) Constipation
      d) Urinary retention
      e) Blurred vision
      f) Tachycardia
      g) Others
   7) Akathesia
   8) Priapism (trazodone)
b. Contraindications/cautionary warnings:
   1) Significant cardiac arrhythmia
   2) Glaucoma (anticholinergic-sensitive, angle closure)
   3) Urinary retention (avoid those with strong anticholinergic effects)
   4) Moderate to severe hypotension
   5) Other
   See standard references for additional untoward reactions, guidelines, contraindications, and warnings.

7. Special considerations

Blood level monitoring is advisable in patients using TCA. The drugs accumulate and have an impact upon cardiac function and lower the seizure threshold. ECG monitoring to evaluate the QRS interval (should be shorter than 100 msec) is recommended. Monitoring liver function is advisable. In patients with a vulnerability toward seizures or when high dosages are required, EEG monitoring is advisable.

TABLE 5.15   **SELECTED ANTIDEPRESSANT DRUGS**[a]

Drug	Noradrenergic-IR[b]	Dopaminergic-IR[b]	Serotonergic-IR[b]	Cholinergic-RA[c]	Histaminic-RA[c]	Adrenergic-RA[c]
Amitriptyline	++++[d]	+	+++	++++	++++	+++
Amoxapine	++	+	++	0	++	+++
Bupropion	0	+++	0	0	0	0
Clomipramine	++	0	++++	++	+	+++
Desipramine	++++	0	++	++	0	+
Fluoxetine	0	0	++++	0	0	0
Imipramine	++	+	+++	++	++	+++
Maprotiline	++++	0	+	+	+++	++
Mianserin	++	++	0	0	+++	+++
Nortriptyline	++++	+	++	++	++	++
Protriptyline	++++	+	++	++++	+	0
Trazodone	0	0	++	0	+	++

[a]Adapted from Warrington SJ, et al. Psychological medicine. Cambridge: Cambridge University Press, 1989.
[b]IR Inhibition of re-uptake
[c]RA Receptor affinity
[d]++++ marked; +++ moderate; ++ minor; + minimal; 0 nil.

D. Antidepressants: Fluoxetine

1. General comments

Fluoxetine is an atypical, nontricyclic antidepressant with potent specific 5–HT reuptake inhibitory properties. It generally has fewer anticholinergic effects than the TCAs, arguably fewer cardiovascular effects, and may cause weight loss. It can be used in combination with TCAs, but combination use results in enhanced blood levels of fluoxetine and the other agent, including anticonvulsants. Toxic responses, including headache, are more likely at high doses, and therefore blood levels should be carefully monitored, particularly in "at-risk" patients, e.g., those with cardiac arrhythmias, seizure disorders, etc.

2. Proposed mechanisms

a. A potent 5–HT reuptake inhibitor
b. Similar mechanism to other antidepressants

3. Recommended use

a. Migraine
b. Daily chronic headache
c. Facial pain syndromes
d. Pain in the presence of psychiatric symptoms that might benefit from the drug

4. Principles of use (see Table 5.21)

Generally, fluoxetine should be initially administered at 20 mg or less per day. Fluoxetine frequently interferes with sleep, even when given early in the day. Gradual increases in dose up to 60–80 mg per day is acceptable, if tolerated. *Synergistic and enhancing effects with other medications occur, and downward dosing of other medications, particularly TCA, phenothiazines, and anticonvulsants, must be considered.*

A syrup form is now available, allowing dosages lower than standard 20 mg capsule size.

5. Drugs in this group

Fluoxetine

6. Selected major untoward reactions and contraindications

a. Untoward reactions

1) Agitation/tremor
2) Nausea
3) Headache
4) Hypomania/delirium/other psychiatric syndromes

5) Insomnia

6) Lower seizure threshold

7) Akathesia/tremor/other extrapyramidal reactions

8) Nausea/diarrhea

9) Anorgasmia/sexual dysfunction

10) Questionable suicidal preoccupation/impulsive behavior

11) Inappropriate secretion of ADH

Unlike some other antidepressants, fluoxetine does not generally cause orthostatic hypotension or cardiac conduction defects. However, fatal reactions have occurred when treatment with MAOIs and fluoxetine has overlapped. *It is strongly recommended that MAOIs be discontinued for at least 3 weeks before fluoxetine is added; fluoxetine should be discontinued for at least 5 weeks before MAOI is added to a treatment regimen.*

Moreover, adverse behavioral and neurological effects have occurred when fluoxetine has been used simultaneously with lithium, haloperidol, tryptophan, or carbamazepine. Because fluoxetine is strongly bound to protein, its use with warfarin and digoxin is of concern, since these drugs may be displaced.

Fluoxetine in combination with other antidepressants or anticonvulsants may have a synergistic or enhancing effect along with increased blood levels. Careful monitoring is necessary. The combined use of fluoxetine and nortriptyline has resulted in seizures even in patients without a previous history. When adding fluoxetine to an existing treatment of other antidepressants or anticonvulsants, it is prudent to reduce the preexisting treatment and then increase both drugs slowly over time, if combined treatment is required.

b. **Selected contraindications/cautionary warnings:**

1) Seizure disorders

2) A strong history of akathesia or extrapyramidal reactions to other antidepressants or phenothiazines

See standard references for additional untoward reactions, guidelines, contraindications, and warnings.

E. Antidepressants: MAO Inhibitors

1. General comments

Monoamine oxidase inhibitors (MAOI) are appropriate for patients with refractory, recurring headache, particularly migraine and certain migraine variant forms. They are similarly helpful in patients with severe depression and headache and are possibly helpful in headache patients with phobic (panic) elements.

Two MAOI subtypes exist:

a. Phenelzine and tranylcypromine preferentially deaminate norepinephrine and 5–HT via inhibition of MAO–A.

b. L–deprenyl preferentially deaminates dopamine via inhibition of MAO–B. (Inhibition of MAO–B has not yet been shown to assist in the control of headache.)

Phenelzine (Nardil) is a nonspecific inhibitor of MAO-A. Phenelzine can be combined with amitriptyline, nortriptyline, and doxepin in cases of refractory headache, but careful and precise administration is required. (See Table 5.16.) *Phenelzine and related agents cannot be combined with imipramine, desipramine, fluoxetine, and several other agents. At least 3 weeks should pass after MAOI discontinuance before these agents are administered. Patients taking MAOIs cannot be safely administered isometheptene (Midrin, Isocom) or meperidine.*

2. Proposed mechanisms

a. Enhancement of synaptic NE and 5–HT
b. Others

3. Recommended use

a. Severe, resistant migraine
b. Severe, resistant, nonneuralgic facial pain syndromes

TABLE 5.16 **GUIDELINES FOR COMBINED MAOI AND TCA USAGE**[a]

1. Begin both phenelzine and TCA (amitriptyline, nortriptyline, or doxepin only) simultaneously, or
2. Add phenelzine to existing program of the above.
3. Do not add TCA to existing treatment of phenelzine.
4. Avoid MAOI usage with imipramine, desipramine, or fluoxetine, and certain others. MAOI must be discontinued for at least 3 weeks before any one of these agents is administered; fluoxetine must be discontinued for at least 5 weeks prior to the administration of MAOI.
5. When switching from one MAOI to another, at least 3 weeks must separate the administration of the second agent from the discontinuation of the first.
6. Informed consent is advisable.

[a]The combined use of MAOI and certain TCA has historically been discouraged. However, this practice is reasonably well established in the treatment of severe, intractable depression. Effective and safe combined usage has been anecdotally reported for a small percentage of patients with severe, intractable headache, some with elements of depression. The reader is strongly advised to employ extreme caution if this program is being considered. Detailed patient education is required. Proper administration is essential and patient selection critical. Avoid use in noncompliant patients or in those who take instruction poorly.

c. Severe, resistant, chronic daily headache and related forms

d. Severe headache in the presence of depression, panic disorder, obsessive-compulsive disorder

4. Principles of use (see Table 5.21)

a. Patients should be placed on a specific MAOI diet in advance of treatment (see Table 5.17) and continue for 3 weeks after discontinuance

b. Patients must carefully adhere to restrictions regarding the use of other drugs, including over-the-counter drugs, cold preparations, etc. (Tables 5.18 and 5.19 may prove helpful.)

5. Selected drugs in this group

a. Phenelzine (Nardil)

b. Tranylcypromine (Parnate)

6. Selected major untoward reactions and contraindications

a. Major untoward reactions

1) Orthostatic hypotension

2) Severe hypertension when combined with a contraindicated drug or food substance

---

TABLE 5.17   **FOODS TO AVOID WHILE ON MAO INHIBITORS**

1. Foods that have a high tyramine content (most common in foods that are aged, fermented, or smoked to increase their flavor), such as cheeses, sour cream, yogurt, pickled herring, chicken livers, bananas, avocadoes, soy sauce, broad bean pods (fava bean pods), yeast extracts, meats prepared with tenderizers, or dry sausage.
2. Alcoholic beverages, including beer and wines (especially Chianti and other hearty red wines).
3. High caffeine-containing foods or beverages, such as coffee, chocolate, tea, or cola.

TABLE 5.18   **SELECTED CATEGORIES OF MEDICATIONS TO BE AVOIDED WITH MAOI**

- Appetite suppressants
- Certain asthma medications
- Decongestant cold medications (including those with dextromethorphan)
- L-tryptophan-containing preparations
- Isometheptene-containing drugs
- Most other antidepressants, particularly fluoxetine, imipramine, desipramine, others
- Mixed allergy drugs (except simple antihistamines)
- Nasal sprays (except steroids only)
- Stimulants and weight-reducing preparations
- Anticonvulsants (specifically carbamazepine)
- Opiate preparations containing meperidine
- Other MAOIs

TABLE 5.19 **SELECTED OVER-THE-COUNTER PRODUCTS CONTAINING EITHER PSEUDOEPHEDRINE, PHENYLEPHRINE, OR PHENYLPROPANOLAMINE**

Pseudoephedrine	
Actifed	Robitussin-PE
Contac	Sine-Aid
CoTylenol	Sinutab
Vicks Formula 44M	Tylenol Maximum Strength
Vicks Formula 44D	Sinus Medication
Vicks Nyquil	
Phenylephrine	
Dimetane Decongestant	Nostril
Dristan Advanced Formula	Vicks Sinex
Tablets and Coated Caplets	Robitussin Night Relief
Neo-Synephrine	
Phenylpropanolamine	
Alka-Seltzer Plus	Coricidin
Acutrim	Dexatrim
Allerest	Sine-Off
Cheracol Plus	Triaminic

  3) Reduced libido (inhibition of ejaculation and/or orgasm)

  4) Constipation

  5) Insomnia

  6) Weight gain

  7) Peripheral edema

  8) Hypomania, agitation

  9) Anticholinergic effects

 b. Contraindications/cautionary warnings

  1) Pheochromocytoma

  2) Certain drugs, among which are:

   a) Fluoxetine

   b) Meperidine (Demerol)

   c) Isometheptene (Midrin)

   d) Carbamazepine

   e) Agents with sympathomimetic effects (decongestants, etc.) (See Tables 5.18 and 5.19)

   f) Pizotofen

  3) Certain foods (see Table 5.17)

  4) Severe liver disease, cardiac disease

  5) Closed angle glaucoma

  6) Severe prostatic disease

  See standard references for additional untoward reactions, guidelines, contraindications, and warnings.

7. Special considerations

  MAOI therapy can be very effective but requires close medical supervision by experienced physicians. Patients must be compliant and well informed. These agents should be administered by physicians with full knowledge of prescribing data who are treating resistant cases of severe headache. Casual use is discouraged.

For severe hypertensive crises, nifedipine (10 mg) should be administered sublingually.

F. Ergot Derivatives: Methysergide, Methylergonovine, Ergonovine Maleate

1. General comments

Currently, these drugs are being used for resistant headache conditions.

Methysergide is the oldest of the prophylactic agents for migraine, cluster, and related headaches. It is effective in migraine prophylaxis in 60% or more of cases.

The historic concern for the development of fibrotic reactions (retroperitoneal fibrosis, pleuropulmonary fibrosis, cardiac valvular changes) after prolonged use of ergot derivatives still exists. However, current belief regarding methysergide is that these responses reflect an *idiosyncratic reaction*, rather than a dose-time-related factor. As such, dose or length of use may not be the primary factor in determining risk.

Ergonovine maleate is no longer commercially available. However, a closely related drug, methylergonovine, which is a metabolite of methysergide, is available as Methergine. The two drug profiles (ergonovine and methylergonovine) are similar and will be considered together. Both are ergot alkaloids. They generally lack the degree of arterial constricting effects of methysergide but have greater oxytotic effects than methysergide or ergotamine tartrate.

2. Proposed mechanisms

a. $5-HT_2$ receptor antagonist
b. $5-HT_1$ agonist
c. Other central effects

3. Recommended use

a. Resistant migraine, including menstrual migraine (episodic prophylaxis)
b. Cluster headache
c. Resistant daily chronic headache
d. Resistant atypical facial pain syndromes

e. Patients placed on these agents should be those in whom more standard medications have failed or could not be used

4. Principles of usage (see Table 5.21)

a. Methysergide
1) 2 mg 3–5 times per day
2) Maximum daily dose is 14 mg per day (preferably 8–10 mg/day)
3) Do not use for more than 6 months without a 1-month interruption and appropriate evaluation for fibrotic reactions

b. Methylergonovine
1) 0.2–0.4 mg t.i.d. to q.i.d.
2) Not advisable to use for more than 6 months without a 1-month interruption and appropriate evaluation for fibrotic reactions

5. Drugs in this group

a. Methysergide (Sansert)
b. Methylergonovine (Methergine)
c. Ergonovine maleate (Ergotrate)

6. Selected major untoward reactions and contraindications

a. Major untoward reactions

1) Nausea
2) Muscle aching (chest, abdomen, legs)
3) Hallucinations
4) Weight gain
5) Frank claudication
6) Fibrotic lesions

In patients using methysergide, fibrotic lesions are estimated to occur in one in 2,000 cases. They have not been reported following the use of ergonovine or methylergonovine.

b. Contraindications/cautionary warnings

1) Peripheral, cerebral, or cardiovascular disease
2) Thrombophlebitis (deep vein)
3) Severe hypertension
4) Pregnancy
5) Significant renal, hepatic disease
6) Previous fibrotic reactions

See standard references for additional untoward reactions, guidelines, contraindications, and warnings.

7. Special considerations

These agents should be administered by physicians who are treating resistant cases of severe headache. A thorough understanding of these drugs is required, and casual use is discouraged.

Most authorities advocate testing for fibrotic reactions at least once every 6 months, during drug holidays. Some authorities believe that if these tests are negative after two to three evaluations, further testing can be reduced considerably. As of yet, this practice is not established as valid or safe.

Patients should generally not be administered these agents continually for more than 6 months without a "drug holiday." However, when serious deterioration of headache control occurs during drug holidays and acceptable alternative treatment is not available, continuous therapy with monitoring may be acceptable. Risk must be carefully explained. Informed consent is advisable.

Table 5.20 provides a recommended evaluation for fibrotic reactions.

G. Anticonvulsants: Phenytoin, Carbamazepine (see next section for valproate)

1. General comments

Anticonvulsants may be effective in the treatment of selected cases of migraine, cluster headache, and facial pain conditions; including true neuralgias and atypical facial pain syndromes. It is not known whether they are more effective in children and adults with paroxysmal EEGs, but at least one report suggests greater efficacy in the presence of disturbed electroencephalographic patterns.

Phenytoin and carbamazepine can reduce the efficacy of oral contraceptives, and therefore specific warnings are necessary.

TABLE 5.20 **RECOMMENDED EVALUATION TO MONITOR FIBROTIC REACTIONS**[a]

1. Cardiac and carotid auscultation for new murmurs or bruits or change from known abnormalities. (Echocardiogram, carotid ultrasound testing recommended if suspected abnormality.)
2. Palpation of peripheral vascular and carotid pulsations. (Ultrasound testing recommended if abnormality suspected.)
3. Abdominal CT scanning (with and without contrast) for retroperitoneal fibrosis.
4. Chest x-ray for pleuropulmonary fibrosis.

[a]Recommended for patients on continuous ergot therapy for 6 months or more.

2. Proposed mechanisms
   a. Membrane stabilization
   b. Possible value in pain control through reduction of paroxysmal discharges

3. Recommended use
   a. Migraine (particularly those associated with paroxysmal EEG patterns)
   b. Cluster headache
   c. Daily chronic headache
   d. Facial pain, atypical facial pain syndromes
   e. Neuralgic syndromes; headache associated with neuralgic features

4. Principles of use (see Table 5.21)
These drugs must be administered carefully, with small divided dosages initially.

Phenytoin is administered in dosages of 200–400 mg per day. Phenytoin in the form of Dilantin can be given as one single dose per day, *but generic forms must be given in divided dosages.*

Carbamazepine (Tegretol) should be given in dosages beginning at 100–200 mg 2–3 times per day, with gradual increase to tolerance or efficacy.

5. Selected major untoward reactions and contraindications
   a. Untoward reactions
     1) Phenytoin: dizziness, drowsiness, rash, insomnia, ataxia, severe drug reactions, etc.
     2) Carbamazepine: leukopenia, dizziness, ataxia, drowsiness, diplopia, severe drug reactions
     3) Concurrent administration with fluoxetine may result in toxicity
     4) Fetal deformity is a significant risk of these drugs
   b. Contraindications/cautionary warnings
     1) Verapamil (and other CAs) potentiates the effects of carbamazepine and perhaps other anticonvulsants
     2) Pregnancy or known allergies to the medication
     3) Oral contraceptive use, unless special warnings are given
     4) Carbamazepine cannot be used concurrently with MAOI
     See standard references for additional untoward reactions, guidelines, contraindications, and warnings.

6. Special considerations

Blood level monitoring is advisable. Also, periodic evaluation for hematological and liver function is recommended, per standard protocol. Inappropriate secretion of ADH has been reported.

Women using oral contraceptives should be warned of possible reduction in efficacy during treatments with these drugs.

H. Anticonvulsants: Valproate

1. General comments

During the past 5 years, there has been increasing interest in valproate as a treatment for headaches. Published studies suggest efficacy, including in otherwise refractory patients.

2. Proposed mechanisms

a. Increased GABA levels in synaptosomes
b. Enhanced postsynaptic response to GABA
c. Increased potassium conductance producing neuronal hyperpolarization
d. Inhibits "firing" of 5–HT neurons of dorsal raphe

3. Recommended use

a. Migraine
b. Daily chronic headache
c. Cluster headache
d. Atypical facial plain syndromes
e. In headache patients with "rapid cycling," bipolar-like illness

4. Principles of use (see Table 5.21)

Valproate should be started at a dose of 125–250 mg 3–4 times per day. A syrup and "sprinkle" form are available. Valproate (Depakote) is available in 125-, 250-, and 500-mg tablet sizes. Optimum effectiveness may occur in serum levels between 50 and 100 μg/ml.

Dosages should be increased gradually to a maximum dosage of 1–2 grams per day.

5. Drugs in this group

Depakote

6. Selected major untoward reactions and contraindications

a. Major untoward reactions

1) Nausea and GI upset
2) Sedation

3) Platelet dysfunction
4) Hair loss
5) Tremor
6) Change in cognition
7) Hepatotoxicity (should be avoided in children unless considered absolutely necessary)
8) Weight gain

In children, hepatic dysfunction with fatal outcome has been reported. The drug is also potentially teratogenic.

b. Contraindications/cautionary warnings:

1) Pregnancy
2) Significant hepatic disease
3) Childhood (relative contraindication. Generally, the drug is inadvisable in patients 10 years of age and below. Very careful monitoring is required if the drug is administered.)
4) Concurrent barbiturate/benzodiazepine use (relative contraindication)
5) Use carefully with other drugs metabolized by the liver

See standard references for additional untoward reactions, guidelines, contraindications, and warnings.

7. Special considerations

It is advisable to evaluate hematological and liver function studies before and during treatment. Blood level monitoring must be carried out periodically. A higher-than-expected potential for adverse effects is present when combined with antidepressants, other anticonvulsants, particularly barbiturates and other liver metabolized drugs, such as verapamil.

Depakote is teratogenic, and accordingly should be used cautiously in fertile women. Warnings are necessary.

Severe sedation and coma have occurred when valproate is combined with barbiturates. In the headache population, strong warning and careful monitoring are necessary because analgesic agents containing barbiturate are frequently prescribed. Because the reaction may be idiosyncratic, risks cannot be predicted or easily anticipated. Some patients are known to be able to use these agents concurrently.

I. Antihistamines (Cyproheptadine, Hydroxyzine)

1. General comments

Antihistamines may be helpful in the symptomatic and preventive treatment of head pain. Historically, cyproheptadine has been used in the preventive treatment of migraine and cluster headache. Hydroxyzine has been used as a symptomatic agent. These drugs are generally considered safe, but sedation, weight gain, and anticholinergic effects have limited their usefulness in some patients.

2. Proposed mechanisms

a. Antagonist at $5-HT_2$ (cyproheptadine)

b. Histamine H_1 and muscarinic receptor influence

c. A primary analgesic effect?

3. Recommended use

a. Migraine (cyproheptadine may be particularly useful in children, symptomatically and preventively)

b. Cluster headache?

c. Atypical facial pain

d. As backup symptomatic medication when analgesics are overused

4. Principles of use

For prevention, small daily dosages should be started, increasing to tolerance or efficacy.

5. Selected drugs in this group

a. Cyproheptadine (Periactin)

b. Hydroxyzine (Vistaril, Atarax)

6. Selected major untoward reactions and contraindications

a. Major untoward reactions

1) Sedation

2) Weight gain

3) Anticholinergic effects

b. Contraindications/cautionary warnings:

1) Closed-angle glaucoma

2) Prostatic hypertrophy

See standard references for additional untoward reactions, guidelines, contraindications, and warnings.

7. Special considerations

These drugs may have special application in children, particularly cyproheptadine. In dosages of 2–4 mg b.i.d. to t.i.d. or 2–4 mg h.s., cyproheptadine may provide effective migraine prophylaxis.

Nighttime sedation may be an added value in some instances.

J. Lithium Carbonate

1. General comments

Lithium carbonate is one of the primary therapies for cluster headache and may have application for other refractory headache conditions as well, including cyclic migraine. It may have added value in patients with migraine and depression, bipolar-like illness, or a family history of bipolar illness.

2. Proposed mechanisms

a. Depletes inositol with resulting dampening of second messenger system

b. Effects on hypothalamus

3. Recommended use

a. Cluster headache

b. Cyclic migraine

c. Atypical facial pain

d. Headache syndromes with significant depression or family history of depression; bipolar or bipolar-like symptoms

4. Principles of use (see Table 5.21)

a. Begin at dosages of 150–300 mg b.i.d. to t.i.d. and titrate upward to b.i.d. to t.i.d.

b. Patients should avoid excessive salt intake (reduces effect) or reduced salt intake (enhances effect).

c. Careful monitoring during periods of increased perspiration (salt loss) is advisable.

d. Blood levels do not correlate with therapeutic benefit for headache but should be monitored to avoid toxicity.

e. Reduce dose when used simultaneously with verapamil and other CAs, and fluoxetine.

f. Monitor thyroid and renal function periodically.

5. Drugs in this group

Various forms of lithium carbonate are available, in slow-release, regular, and syrup form.

6. Selected major untoward reactions and contraindications

a. Major untoward reactions

1) Tremor/imbalance

2) Polyuria

3) Thirst

4) Edema

5) Mental changes

6) Increase in white blood count (leukocytosis)

Long-term usage may induce hypothyroidism, oliguric renal failure, and diabetes insipidus.

Careful monitoring when used with calcium antagonists is required. Toxic effects of lithium may appear despite normal serum levels and at standard lithium doses when concurrently used with CA or fluoxetine. Concurrent use with diuretics is not advisable, since sodium depletion or renal changes are possible.

b. Contraindications/cautionary warnings

1) Significant renal or cardiovascular disease

2) Dehydration

3) Sodium depletion

4) Hypothyroidism

See standard references for additional untoward reactions, guidelines, contraindications, and warnings.

K. Pizotofen (Sandomigrin)

1. General comments

Pizotofen is not available in the U.S. but is widely used in Canada. It is reported to be of significant value in patients with migraine.

2. Proposed mechanisms

a. 5–HT receptor agonist

b. Similar to that of cyproheptadine

3. Recommended use

a. Migraine

b. Cluster headache

4. Principles of use

The drug is started at 0.5 mg at h.s., gradually increasing to 0.5 mg t.i.d. The entire dose can be given at night, up to 6 mg per day.

5. Drugs in this group

Sandomigran

6. Selected major untoward reactions and contraindications

Untoward reactions include drowsiness and weight gain. Contraindications include patients simultaneously using MAOIs or within 3 weeks of MAOI discontinuance.

See standard references for additional untoward reactions, guidelines, contraindications, and warnings.

L. Other Drugs
1. Captopril

Captopril, an angiotensin-converting enzyme (ACE) inhibitor, has been suggested as effective in migraine patients. The mechanism by which it may control migraine is unknown. Dosing begins with 12.5–25 mg b.i.d., gradually increasing in divided dosages to approximately 150 mg per day, if untoward reactions do not prohibit further usage.

Proteinuria, hypotension, angioedema, skin rash, and loss of taste are possible. Cough occurs in 5–20% of patients. Teratogenic effects are a recently reported concern.

See standard references for additional untoward reactions, guidelines, contraindications, and warnings.

2. Clonidine

Clonidine, an activator of α-2-adrenergic receptors, has been reported to be of use by stimulating presynaptic inhibitory α-2-receptors. It may have particular value in treating withdrawal symptoms from narcotics in headache patients and may enhance the analgesic effects of opiates. Its specific value for headache remains debatable. Nicotine withdrawal symptomatology may be similarly reduced with clonidine treatment.

Clonidine is available in various forms. In addition to tablets of 0.1 mg, 0.2 mg, and 0.3 mg, Catapres patches deliver 0.1, 0.2, or 0.3 mg per day of the drug.

Major untoward reactions include dry mouth, drowsiness, dizziness, constipation, and sedation. *When used simultaneously with β-adrenergic blockers, careful reduction of either agent is required, since hypertensive reactions are possible.*

See standard references for additional untoward reactions, guidelines, contraindications, and warnings.

3. Baclofen

Baclofen (Lioresal) is a muscle relaxant and antispasmodic, the precise mechanism of action of which is unknown. It inhibits both monosynaptic and polysynaptic reflexes at the spinal level, is an analogue of the putative inhibitory neurotransmitter γ-aminobutyric acid (GABA), and has central CNS depressant properties, including sedation, somnolence, ataxia, and respiratory and cardiovascular depression.

In pain treatment, baclofen is of greatest value in the treatment of neuralgic syndromes. It may be added to other antineuralgic therapies, administered 10 mg b.i.d. to t.i.d., with upward titration to 60–80 mg per day. Tolerance usually develops to its untoward reactions, but very slow, upward dosing is recommended.

See standard references for additional untoward reactions, guidelines, contraindications, and warnings.

4. Muscle relaxants

A variety of other "muscle relaxants" are available and have anecdotal value in the treatment of headache. Most of these drugs, such as metaxalone (Skelaxin), have central actions that may be the mechanism by which they reduce head pain, symptomatically and preventively.

See standard references for additional untoward reactions, guidelines, contraindications, and warnings.

5. Caffeine sodium benzoate

Caffeine sodium benzoate may be of value in the treatment of low CSF pressure headache, such as following a spinal tap or in spontaneous low-pressure syndromes (see Chapter 15). A dose of 0.5 grams (500 mg) is given intravenously in one of several regimens:

- An ampule (500 mg) may be added to D–5 lactated Ringer's solution (500–1000 ml) and administered over several hours or longer; and
- An ampule (500 mg) administered via a syringe containing 25 mg of normal saline by "slow push."

Careful monitoring for palpitations and other effects of caffeine is required.

See standard references for additional untoward reactions, guidelines, contraindications, and warnings.

M. Capsaicin

Capsaicin, the active ingredient of hot peppers, selectively diminishes sensations of heat pain and neurogenic vasodilation by desensitizing unmyelinated/C-fiber nociceptors. Evidence is accumulating that it may be effective in controlling the pain of diabetic neuropathy, postherpetic neuralgia, causalgia, reflex sympathetic dystrophy, and other disorders of the peripheral nerve. Concentrations of 0.025% and 0.075% are available.

TABLE 5.21. SELECTED DRUGS USED IN THE PHARMACOTHERAPY OF HEAD, NECK AND FACE PAIN

Drug Name	Mg/Dose	Standard Daily Admin.	Notes
Symptomatic treatment			
ANALGESICS[a]			
NSAIDs	—	varies	Avoid more than 2 days/wk of use
Naproxen sodium[a] (p.o.)	275–550	bid–tid	Avoid extended, daily use
Indomethacin[a] (p.o.)	25–50	bid–tid	Avoid extended, daily use
Indocin SR	75	1 q day or bid	Avoid extended, daily use
Indomethacin supp	50	bid–tid	Avoid extended, daily use
Meclofenamate[a] (p.o.)	50–200	bid	Avoid extended, daily use
Ibuprofen[a] (p.o.)	600–800	bid–tid	Avoid extended, daily use
Ketorolac[a] (p.o.)	10	qid	Avoid extended, daily use
Ketorolac (IM)	30–60	tid	Appears particularly valuable when ergot derivatives and narcotics must be avoided and parenteral therapy is necessary
SPECIAL MIGRAINE DRUGS			
Isometheptene[a] combinations (Midrin, etc.)	—	2 tabs at onset; 1–2 q 30–60 min.	Max 5–6 tabs/day; 2 days/wk
Ergotamine tartrate (ET)			
Oral (Cafergot Wigraine, etc.)[a]	1 mg ET, 100 mg caffeine	2 tabs at onset; 1–2 q 30–60 min	Max 4–6/day; 2 days/wk
Suppositories (Cafergot, Wigraine)	2 mg ET, 100 mg caffeine	1/3–1 at onset; may repeat in 60 min × 1	Max 2/day; 2 days/wk
Sublingual (Ergomar, Ergostat)	2 mg ET	1 at onset may repeat after 15 min × 1	Max 2/day; 2 days/wk
Dihydroergotamine (DHE)			
Intramuscular	0.25–1 mg	0.25–1 mg SC, IM tid	Can be used 2–3 times/day in conjunction with antinauseant, analgesic, etc. IM more effective than SC. Fig. 5.1, Table 5.6.
Intravenous	" "	See protocols in text, Chapters 5 and 6	
PHENOTHIAZINE/NEUROLEPTIC			
Chlorpromazine			
(p.o.)[a]	25–100	bid–tid	Limit 3 days/wk; avoid extended use
(supp)	25–100	bid–tid	Limit 3 days/wk; avoid extended use

(IM)	25–100	bid–tid	Limit 3 days/wk; avoid extended use
(IV)	—	—	See Chapter 6
Metoclopramide			
p.o. (tablet and syrup)	10–20	tid	Limit 3 days/wk; avoid extended use
parenteral	10–15	tid	Limit 3 days/wk; avoid extended use
Promethazine			
(p.o.)	25–75	tid	Limit 3 days/wk; avoid extended use
(IM)	25–75	tid	Limit 3 days/wk; avoid extended use
Perphenazine			
(p.o.)	2–4	bid–tid	Limit 3 days/wk; avoid extended use
(IM)	5	bid	Limit 3 days/wk; avoid extended use
ANTIHISTAMINES			
Hydroxyzine (p.o.)	50–100	bid–tid or at hs	Can be used as a symptomatic treatment
Cyproheptadine (p.o.)	2–4	tid–qid or at hs	Can be used as a symptomatic treatment
STEROIDS			
Prednisone	40–60	in 1 or divided doses	4–10 day program. Avoid repeated use.
Hydrocortisone (IV)			See Chapter 6
Preventive Drugs[b]			
TRICYCLIC ANTIDEPRESSANTS (see Table 5.15)			
Amitriptyline	10–150	Divided doses or hs	Bedtime dose aids sleep disturbance
Nortriptyline	10–100	Divided doses or hs	Bedtime dose aids sleep disturbance
Doxepin	10–150	Divided doses or hs	Bedtime dose aids sleep disturbance
OTHER ANTIDEPRESSANTS			
Fluoxetine	20	20–80 mg/day in divided dose	Efficacy under study; minimal sedation
MAO INHIBITORS[c]			
Phenelzine	15–30	15–60 mg/day in divided dose	Dietary and medicine restrictions mandatory; (see appropriate tables)
β-ADRENERGIC BLOCKERS (see Table 5.15)			
Propranolol	20–80	tid–qid (standard form)	Monitor cardiac function, BP, pulse, lipids
Inderal LA	80–160	bid	Monitor cardiac function, BP, pulse, lipids
Atenolol	50–100	bid	Monitor cardiac function, BP, pulse, lipids
Timolol	10–20	bid	Monitor cardiac function, BP, pulse, lipids
Metoprolol	50–100	bid	Monitor cardiac function, BP, pulse, lipids
Nadolol	20–120	bid	Monitor cardiac function, BP, pulse, lipids; Metabolized by kidneys

TABLE 5.21. **CONTINUED**

Drug Name	Mg/Dose	Standard Daily Admin.	Notes
CALCIUM CHANNEL BLOCKERS			
Verapamil	80–160	tid–qid	Monitor cardiac function, BP, pulse
Nimodipine	30–60	tid	Monitor cardiac function, BP, pulse
Diltiazam	30–90	tid	Monitor cardiac function, BP, pulse
Nifedipine	10–30	tid	Monitor cardiac function, BP, pulse. Sublingual for severe hypertensive reactions or intense neural symptoms with migraine
ERGOTAMINE DERIVATIVES			
Methysergide	1–2	tid–5×/day	After 6-month treatment, review cardiac, pulmonary, and retroperitoneal regions for fibrotic changes. Carefully observe contraindications
Methylergonovine/ergonovine maleate	0.2–0.4	tid–qid	After 6-month treatment, review cardiac, pulmonary, and retroperitoneal regions for fibrotic changes. Carefully observe contraindications
ANTICONVULSANTS			
Valproate	125–500	1–2 g/day in divided dosages	Monitor hepatic and metabolic parameters carefully. Consider dose reduction when used with antidepressants, lithium, verapamil, phenothiazines, other anticonvulsants. Observe warnings carefully

Carbamazepine	100–200	300–1200 mg/day in divided doses	Monitor hepatic and metabolic parameters carefully. Consider dose reduction when used with antidepressants, lithium, verapamil, phenothiazines, other anticonvulsants. Observe warnings carefully. Reduces oral contraceptive efficacy
Phenytoin	100–300	300–400 mg/day in divided doses or single daily dose[d]	Monitor hepatic and metabolic parameters carefully. Consider dose reduction when used with antidepressants, lithium, verapamil, phenothiazines, other anticonvulsants. Observe warnings carefully. Reduces oral contraceptive efficacy
OTHERS			
Baclofen (Lioresal)	10–20	tid–qid	Increase dose slowly and allow tolerance to develop
Sodium caffeine benzoate	0.5 g (500 mg)	1–2 ampules/day	See text for discussion on administration
Lithium	150–300	bid–tid	Reduce dose in conjunction with verapamil and other calcium antagonists; monitor metabolic parameters
Oxygen inhalation	100% O_2 with mask	7 liters/min for 10–15 min	Must be used at onset of attack of cluster headache; avoid around extreme heat or flame, such as cigarettes

[a] Oral absorption often impaired in migraine; may require alternate route or facilitation with oral metoclopramide administered 1/2 hour before headache medication.
[b] Avoid sustained use of preventive medication for more than 6 months without trial reduction.
[c] Can be combined with certain tricyclic antidepressants, such as amitriptyline, nortriptyline, and doxepin.
[d] Dilantin Kapseals can be given as a single daily dose. This is not the case with generic form of phenytoin.

TABLE 5.22 **SELECTED SYMPTOMATIC MEDICATION GROUPS FOR HEADACHE AND FACIAL PAIN BY ROUTE OF ADMINISTRATION**

Oral	Rectal	Parenteral
Analgesics	Ergotamine tartrate	Analgesics
Over the-Counter	Phenothiazines	Narcotic
NSAIDs	Chlorpromazine	Agonist-antagonist
Naproxen sodium	Prochlorperazine	DHE
Indomethacin	Indomethacin	Ketorolac
Meclofenamate	Morphine sulfate	Phenothiazines
Mixed analgesics		Hydroxyzine
Fiorinal		Steroids (hydrocortisone)
Fiorinal w/codeine		Sumatriptan
Fioricet		
Tylenol w/codeine		
Vicodin (hydrocodone)		
Percocet (oxycodone)		
Specific Migraine Drugs		
Ergotamine tartrate		
Isometheptene		
Sumatriptan		
Phenothiazines/		
antihistamines		
Chlorpromazine		
Perfenazine		
Hydroxyzine		
Steroids		
Prednisone		
Dexamethasone		

TABLE 5.23. **SELECTED WARNINGS ON INTERACTIONS OF COMMONLY USED HEADACHE MEDICATION COMBINATIONS**

Drugs	Warnings
Lithium and verapamil/CCA[a]	Lithium toxicity potentiated
Depakote and TCA, fluoxetine	Enhanced Depakote effects, potential liver toxicity
Depakote and barbiturate (? benzodiazepine)	Idiosyncratic sedation/coma
Anticonvulsant (except valproate) and oral contraceptives	Reduced efficacy of oral contraceptives
MAOI with most TCAs	Serotonin syndrome/hypertensive crisis
MAOI and isometheptene	Hypertensive crisis
MAOI and meperidine	Stimulant reaction, sudden death
MAOI and fluoxetine	Serotonin syndrome, sudden death
MAOI and carbamazepine	Hypertensive crisis
Fluoxetine and phenothiazine	Enhanced extrapyramidal effects
Fluoxetine and MAOI	Serotonin syndromes/sudden death
Fluoxetine and lithium	Potentiates lithium toxicity
CCA[a] and anticonvulsants	Enhanced anticonvulsant effect
CCA[a] and lithium	Potentiates lithium toxicity

[a]Calcium channel antagonists.

6

Treatment of Intractable, Severe Migraine
Matching the Intensity of Treatment to the Severity of Illness

I. Introduction, Definition, and Overview

Acute, periodic migraine is defined as a severe migraine headache that is usually self-limited (less than 72 hours) if untreated. Although generally responsive to self-administered treatments, occasionally the attack is either unresponsive to self-treatment and/or accompanied by such intense pain, nausea, and vomiting that acute care intervention is mandatory.

Acute, intractable (persistent, progressive) migraine is defined as a sustained (persistent, nonself-limited), severe migraine and accompaniments, which are not effectively terminated (sustained control) by appropriate outpatient interventions. This condition generally requires continuing acute therapeutic treatments over a day or longer, sometimes as much as 8–10 days. The illness is similar to that which has been historically referred to as *status migrainosis*. Patients can be severely incapacitated and at risk if the condition is protracted.

A. Clinical Features of *Acute, Intractable Migraine*

1. Continuing, persistent, severe head, neck, or face pain
2. Progressive physical and emotional accompaniments, which may include:
   a. Nausea, vomiting, and diarrhea
   b. Dehydration
   c. Despair/depression
   d. Alteration of normal sleeping, eating, and activities of daily living
   e. Additional migraine accompaniments: Photo- and phonosensitivity, malaise, focal neurological symptoms, etc.
3. Toxicity and/or withdrawal symptoms from excessive use of symptomatic medication, with or without a history of dependency/addiction

B. Treatment Overview

Treatment of *Acute, Periodic Migraine* and *Intractable Migraine* departs markedly from the treatment of more ordinary headache events. Patients with these severe states of pain require aggressive intervention, which usually mandates one or more of the following:

1. Parenteral pain therapy
2. Rehydration
3. Control of nausea and vomiting
4. Removal of provoking factors, including medications
5. Support (psychological and physiological)
6. Monitoring in an acute care setting

   The principal challenge to effective treatment is to match the intensity of treatment to the severity of illness.

C. Other Considerations

1. Patients with *acute, intractable migraine syndromes* suffer the often escalating consequences of head pain *plus* accompaniments, some of which are more serious and debilitating than the headache itself. In the presence of toxic medication effects or "rebound" dependency (see later), withdrawal symptomatology is likely when overused, addictive, symptomatic medications are withdrawn.

2. If present, dehydration may result from a combination of factors, including:

   a. Reduced fluid intake over days or weeks

   b. Increased fluid and electrolyte loss through emesis, diarrhea,

      and polyuria

   c. Diaphoresis

II. Contributing Factors to Acute, Intractable Migraine

The following are considered factors that might contribute to the intractable headache status.

A. Drug-related Causes

1. The *rebound phenomenon*, as described in Chapter 5 and Chapter 7, is a self-sustaining condition, characterized by a persisting and recurring headache against a background of chronic and regular use of a centrally acting analgesic or ergot derivative capable of producing this medication/ headache cycle. Generally, patients will undergo weeks, months, or even years of excessive use of centrally acting analgesics or ergot derivatives prior to the presentation. Attempts to withdraw or discontinue the overused medications result in a dramatic escalation of pain, prompting physician readministration or desperate attempts to obtain medication for self-administration.

2. In addition to the "rebound effect," which reflects both physiological and psychological dependence, toxic symp-

toms (including headache) can result from excessive use of certain drugs (caffeine, ergot preparations, opiates, acetaminophen, etc.), thereby further contributing to the intractable state.

Removal of the offending agent(s) is critical to establishing effective treatment. Patients are refractory to standard treatments during active phases of the rebound phenomenon. Successful discontinuance may itself result in a substantial reduction in the frequency of headache, although initially a marked increase in headache intensity may occur (the rebound effect) before improvement is achieved.

B. Endocrine Disturbances

Endocrine factors, including estrogen replacement or the use of oral contraceptives, for example, may contribute to prolonged, protracted migraine.

C. The Presence of Disease

The presence of comorbid intracranial, cranial, cervical, or systemic disease, particularly if the peripheral pathways of the trigeminal system or the occipitocervical junction are involved, can be a major factor contributing to acute, intractable headache.

D. Head Injury

E. Severe, Intense Psychological Duress

F. *Intractable Migraine* without Apparent Causes

Intractable migraine occasionally develops without apparent aggravating influence.

III. Choosing the Proper Setting for Treatment

Patients with *acute, intractable migraine* may sometimes benefit from aggressive outpatient services, including emergency department therapy, but frequently require hospitalization for acute treatment.

A. Emergency Services—Appropriate

Emergency department service is appropriate in the following circumstances:

1. To treat moderate to severe headache, *unaccompanied* by drug toxicity, dependency, or rebound, and which is likely to abate after a single treatment
2. To rapidly rule out accompanying severe neurological or medical illness (subarachnoid hemorrhage, etc.)
3. When headaches are associated with a suicidal potential (suicidal risk evaluation is necessary)

B. Emergency Services—Inappropriate

Emergency department service are less suitable when headaches are accompanied by:

1. Dehydration, electrolyte depletion, and/or hypotension, which require prolonged therapy or sustained monitoring
2. Toxic/rebound or dependency states, requiring days to weeks to resolve
3. Intractable nausea, vomiting, or diarrhea, requiring many hours or days to treat and which may recur
4. Concurrent medical illness influencing or limiting the effective treatment of headache
5. The likelihood of delayed withdrawal phenomena, with potential for marked increase in pain, seizures, diarrhea, leg and abdominal cramps, etc.
6. A pattern of multiple emergency department treatments
7. The likelihood that emergency services will not be able to address the headache patient's needs promptly and effectively

Although emergency department treatment for acute headache is improving, historically it has been suboptimal. Cynicism and delay in treatment still characterize the experience of many headache patients in emergency departments, no matter how ill they are. While narcotic administration may be appropriate in certain circumstances, reliance on narcotic analgesics alone is often the mainstay of treatment in emergency department settings, despite the availability of more appropriate and specific agents, such as dihydroergotamine (DHE), parenteral phenothiazines, and other agents.

C. Criteria for Hospitalization

The following are among the criteria justifying admission to the hospital or a similar acute care setting. (These are modified from admission criteria established jointly by the Michigan Head·Pain & Neurological Institute in Ann Arbor and Blue Cross/Blue Shield of Michigan):

1. Moderate to severe, intractable headache failing to respond to appropriate and aggressive outpatient or emergency department measures and requiring repetitive, sustained parenteral treatment (e.g., DHE, etc.)
2. The presence of continuing nausea, vomiting, or diarrhea
3. The need to detoxify and treat toxicity, dependency, or rebound phenomena and/or monitor carefully against withdrawal symptoms, including seizures
4. The presence of dehydration, electrolyte imbalance, and prostration, requiring monitoring and intravenous fluids
5. The presence of unstable vital signs
6. The presence of repeated, previous emergency department treatments

7. The likely presence of serious disease (e.g., SAH, intracranial infection, cerebral ischemia, severe hypertension, etc.)

8. The need to simultaneously develop an effective pharmacological prophylaxis in order to sustain improvement achieved by parenteral therapy (aggressive daily drug manipulation, requiring careful monitoring and drug level evaluation)

9. The need to acutely address other comorbid conditions contributing to or accompanying the headache, including medical or psychological illness

10. Concurrent medical and/or psychological illnesses requiring careful monitoring in high-risk situations

D. Clinical Variables That Determine Treatment Setting

The following clinical variables and conditions can be used to determine the most appropriate setting for care:

1. The intensity and duration of pain

2. The presence and degree of toxicity, "rebound," or dependency (physiological and/or psychological)

3. The addiction potential of excessively used drugs (predicts the difficulty of discontinuance and likelihood of withdrawal symptoms)

4. The patient's drug dependency profile

5. Capacity of the patient to cope with pain on an outpatient basis as treatment trials are undertaken

6. Anticipated difficulty of establishing a preventive program

7. Need for supportive measures
   a. Fluids
   b. Repetitive parenteral pain control treatment
   c. Treatment of withdrawal symptoms (nausea and vomiting, seizures with barbiturate withdrawal, muscle cramps, diarrhea, and abdominal pain from narcotic withdrawal, etc.)

8. The presence of complicating medical problems, including
   a. Cardiac disease
   b. Seizure disorders
   c. Hypertension
   d. Peripheral vascular disorders
   e. Others

9. General psychological and physiological health factors

IV. Protocols for Managing Acute, Intractable Migraine
A. Emergency Department Setting

In an emergency department setting (for occasional, periodic, uncomplicated attacks of prolonged migraine):

1. General measures: vital signs, rule out comorbid disease, ECG, etc.

2. Parenteral treatments

    a. Intramuscular or intravenous DHE (see protocol)

    b. Ketorolac

    c. Narcotics

    d. Intravenous phenothiazine (see protocol)

    e. Antiemetics

    f. Others (sumatriptan if and when available)

B. Inpatient Setting

In an inpatient setting (hospital) for protracted, complicated, disabling attacks:

1. General guidelines:

    a. Replace fluids and electrolytes; carefully monitor for dehydration

    b. Treat nausea, vomiting, and diarrhea; control blood pressure if necessary

    c. Discontinue offending medications (if withdrawal is likely, appropriate measures should be undertaken)

    d. Implement acute parenteral pain management (see below)

    e. When appropriate, gradually implement preventive measures to achieve pain control after acute care is terminated

    f. Identify appropriate outpatient symptomatic treatments for use after discharge

    g. Instruct patient and family in the use of treatments and self-help measures to avoid future hospitalizations

    h. When appropriate, psychological and behavioral evaluation and treatment, family counseling, drug overuse treatment, etc.

2. Parenteral protocols

    a. General measures

        1) Inform patient of procedure, risks, and advantages

        2) Establish baseline vital signs

        3) Perform and review baseline electrocardiogram

        4) Establish peripheral IV access

        5) Consider administering "piggy-back" or have available IV fluids for emergency needs

6) Following administration, monitor vital signs during the first hour and as appropriate thereafter
7) Establish availability of emergency equipment and personnel
  b. Specific protocols
    1) Intravenous DHE (see Table 6.1; Figure 6.1)
    2) Intravenous phenothiazines
      a. Chlorpromazine
        i. 7.5–20 mg chlorpromazine (Thorazine)
        ii. In 25–50 cc saline "drip" or slow "push" (over 2 minutes)
        iii. b.i.d.–t.i.d.; administer as needed
            Monitor carefully for orthostatic hypotension and other adverse effects for several hours after administration. Administer IV diphenhydramine if acute dystonic reactions occur.
      b. Prochlorperazine (Compazine)
        i. 10 mg prochlorperazine (Compazine)
        ii. In 25–50 cc saline "drip" or slow "push" (over 2 minutes)

TABLE 6.1 **INTRAVENOUS PROTOCOL FOR DIHYDROERGOTAMINE ADMINISTRATION (See also Table 5.6)**

A. Protocol
  1. 0.25–0.5 mg IV "push" (test dose), over 2 minutes via heparin lock apparatus. (Do not administer in presence of moderate or greater hypertension.)
  2. If tolerated, DHE 0.5–1 mg IV "push" q 8 hours.
  3. Administer 10 mg metoclopramide (IV[a] or IM) before DHE administration, if nausea occurs.
  4. Maintain for 3–5 days, if tolerated. May repeat program one time.
B. Guidelines for Use
  1. Administer metoclopramide before or with DHE administration if necessary to control nausea. Discontinue if not necessary.
  2. DHE to be administered via 1–2 minute slow "push."
  3. Most patients stabilize at end of day 3, but extension of program for 2–3 more days may be necessary.
  4. Discontinue DHE via a 1–3 day gradual reduction program if patient is pain-free for 2 days.
  5. Hospitalization is most appropriate for sustained therapy, during which careful monitoring for blood pressure elevation, chest pain, severe nausea, etc. can be carried out and necessary concurrent therapies can be administered, including establishment of an effective preventive program.
  6. Discontinue or substantially reduce dose if significant elevation of blood pressure, severe nausea, chest pain, severe leg cramps, or other significant adverse reactions occur.

[a]10 mg slow "IV push" or in 50 cc 5% dextrose in water (D5W) over 20–30 minutes.

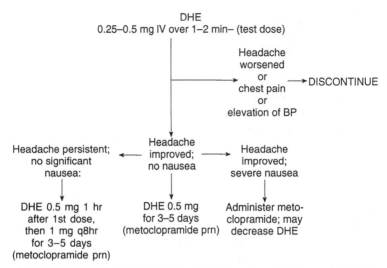

When discounting after several days' use, reduce the dose gradually over a day or so.

Figure 6.1. Algorithm for IV DHE administration.

   iii. b.i.d.–t.i.d.; administer as needed
     Monitor carefully for orthostatic hypotension and other adverse effects for several hours after administration. Administer IV diphenhydramine if acute dystonic reactions occur.

  3) Hydrocortisone
  a. 100 mg hydrocortisone intravenous "push" (2 cc)
  b. q 6 hr for 24 hr
  c. q 8 hr for 24 hr
  d. q 12 hr for 24 hr

  This drug should be used restrictively because of potential adverse events, including avascular necrosis of bone. The clinical need, total amount of steroids previously administered, as well as frequency of use are important considerations in determining usage and length of administration. Carefully review for the presence of infection and other contraindications.

  4) Parenteral ketorolac
  a. 30–60 mg IM t.i.d.
  b. 3–5 day regimen for intractable headache

VI. Comprehensive Centers
A. Introduction
  Though comprehensive, multidisciplinary intervention is not available in most locations, this intensive treatment for dif-

ficult and complex patients has been shown to have an important care and cost-effective value for appropriately chosen patients. Outcome studies from the Michigan Head·Pain & Neurological Institute in Ann Arbor and its affiliated inpatient unit at Chelsea Community Hospital in Chelsea, Michigan have shown a sustained and noteworthy reduction in pain, depression, symptomatic drug use, and emergency room utilization, along with a return to work in an impressive number of patients who had been disabled prior to treatment (Lake and Saper, 1990). This study was a 2-year prospective analysis of patients admitted to the hospital treatment unit (also see Silberstein, 1992).

B. Criteria for Referral to a Comprehensive Center for Headache Management

1. History of recurring acute care needs or progressive, persistent headache
2. Multiple diagnostic and therapeutic interventions by qualified physicians without successful outcome
3. Evidence of excessive utilization of outpatient services, diagnostic procedures, or repeated hospital admissions for narcotic analgesics or other parenteral treatments
4. Uncertain or questionable diagnosis
5. When comprehensive, multidisciplinary services are essential to address the multifactorial components of pain

SPECIFIC CONDITIONS
Introduction to Chapters 7–17

The following chapters will profile the primary headache disorders and selected clinical entities, including the neuralgias, atypical facial pain disorders, and several organic/metabolic conditions. The chapters are not meant to provide exhaustive reviews but to highlight practical considerations of each condition, with recommendations for diagnostic evaluation and treatment.

Details of pharmacotherapy, as recommended under the treatment sections in each chapter, can be found in Chapters 5 and 6. Diagnostic testing is described in Chapter 2.

7

Migraine

I. Introduction

Migraine embodies a large number of headache presentations, ranging from typical, characteristic attacks to many variant forms. It includes, in our opinion, what has traditionally been called "ordinary" or minor headache and so-called *tension headache* (see Chapter 8). In practice, what has been called *acute tension headache* and is now called *episodic tension-type headache* is largely indistinguishable symptomatically and therapeutically from episodic migraine.

In its typical form, migraine is a complex neurophysiological disorder characterized by episodic and, in its progressive form, daily head pain. The headache attacks are often accompanied by neurological, autonomic, and psychophysiological events. Seventy-six percent of women and 57% of men suffer from recurring headache. We believe most suffer from a form of migraine.

Formerly, migraine was divided into two major subgroups: *classic* and *common* migraine. *Classic migraine* is now called (IHS classification) *migraine with aura*, and *common migraine* is called *migraine without aura*. (See Table 7.1, 7.2)

Approximately 30% of migraine attacks are "with aura." Many patients have both forms. The aura of migraine may precede, accompany, or follow the actual headache attack.

Since the late 1970s, there has been increasing recognition of migraine's capacity to *transform* from intermittent attacks to daily or almost daily head pain. This "variant" form of migraine, which has been termed *transformational migraine, progressive migraine, or pernicious migraine*, represents a progressive form of the illness in which, for uncertain reasons, intermittent migraine attacks increase in frequency, eventually transforming into continuous headache, with periodic, attacks of acute migraine superimposed.

II. Key Clinical Features

Generally, migraine is an inherited disorder. An autosomal dominant trait with incomplete penetrance has been proposed. Sex distribution is approximately equal in childhood. But adult migraine affects women in a ratio of approximately 3:1 to males.

TABLE 7.1. **NEW INTERNATIONAL HEADACHE SOCIETY DEFINITION OF MIGRAINE WITHOUT AURA**[a]

1.1 *Migraine without aura*
Previously used terms: common migraine, hemicrania simplex
Diagnostic criteria:
A. At least five attacks fulfilling B-D
B. Headache lasting 4 to 72 hours (untreated or unsuccessfully treated)
C. Headache has at least two of the following characteristics:
   1. Unilateral location
   2. Pulsating quality
   3. Moderate or severe intensity (inhibits or prohibits daily activities)
   4. Aggravation by walking stairs or similar routine physical activity
D. During headache at least one of the following:
   1. Nausea and/or vomiting
   2. Photophobia and phonophobia
E. At least one of the following:
   1. History, physical, and neurological examinations do not suggest one of the disorders listed in groups 5–11 (see reference below)
   2. History and/or physical and/or neurological examinations do suggest such disorder, but it is ruled out by appropriate investigations
   3. Such disorder is present, but migraine attacks do not occur for the first time in close temporal relation to the disorder

[a]From Headache Classification Committee of the International Headache Society. Classification and diagnostic criteria for headache disorders, cranial neuralgias, and facial pain. Cephalalgia 1988; 8 (Suppl 7): 1–96.

This dominance reflects the aggravating influence of *estrogen* on the migraine mechanism and the generally better prognosis of childhood migraine in males. Most patients develop migraine in the first three decades of life, but it can develop for the first time during any decade.

The following phases of migraine are recognized and may occur alone or in combination with any other phase.

A. The Prodrome

The prodrome is a set of premonitory phenomena generally occurring hours to days before the headache, and consisting of mental, nonspecific neurological, constitutional, or autonomic symptoms. Neurological phenomena, such as photophobia and phonophobia (increased sensitivity to light and sound, respectively) and hyperosmia (increased sensitivity to smells), are common.

Table 7.3 lists selected prodromal features of migraine.

The presence of stiff neck as part of the prodrome has led many to consider erroneously "tension headache" or cervical pathology as the origin of the complaint.

B. The Aura

The *aura* is comprised of focal neurological symptoms that usually precede the headache by 5–20 minutes. Less

TABLE 7.2. **NEW INTERNATIONAL HEADACHE SOCIETY DEFINITION OF MIGRAINE WITH AURA**[a]

1.2 *Migraine with aura*
Previously used terms: classic migraine, classical migraine, ophthalmic, hemiparesthetic, hemiplegic, or aphasic migraine
Diagnostic criteria:
A. At least two attacks fulfilling B
B. At least three of the following four characteristics:
   1. One or more fully reversible aura symptoms indicating focal cerebral cortical and/or brainstem dysfunction
   2. At least one aura symptom develops gradually over more than 4 minutes or two or more symptoms occur in succession
   3. No aura symptom lasts more than 60 minutes. If more than one aura symptom is present, accepted duration is proportionally increased
   4. Headache follows aura with a free interval of less than 60 minutes. (It may also begin before or simultaneously with the aura)
C. At least one of the following:
   1. History, physical, and neurological examinations do not suggest one of the disorders listed in groups 5–11 (see reference below)
   2. History and/or physical and/or neurological examinations do suggest such disorder, but it is ruled out by appropriate investigations
   3. Such disorder is present, but migraine attacks do not occur for the first time in close temporal relation to the disorder
1.2.1 *Migraine with typical aura*
Diagnostic criteria:
A. Fulfills criteria for 1.2 including all four criteria under B
B. One or more aura symptoms of the following types:
   1. Homonymous visual disturbance
   2. Unilateral paresthesias and/or numbness
   3. Unilateral weakness
   4. Aphasia or unclassifiable speech difficulty

[a]From Headache Classification Committee of the International Headache Society. Classification and Diagnostic criteria for headache disorders, cranial neuralgias, and facial pains. Cephalalgia 1988; 8 (Suppl 7): 1–96.

TABLE 7.3. **SELECTED PRODROMAL FEATURES OF MIGRAINE**

Mental and mood changes (depression, anger, euphoria, hypomania, etc.)
Stiff neck
A chilled feeling, peripheral vasoconstriction
Sluggishness/fatigue/excessive tiredness/yawning
Increased frequency of urination
Anorexia
Constipation or diarrhea
Fluid retention
Food cravings

often, the aura may begin simultaneously with the headache phase or after it has begun. The aura may occur alone, not accompanied or followed by a subsequent headache. If the aura is prolonged, it may meet the criteria established for *complicated* or *hemiplegic migraine* (see later).

The most common symptoms of the aura are visual, particularly *fortification spectra*, which are zigzag or scintillating images.

Table 7.4 lists selected features of the aura.

C. The Headache

The headache of migraine may be unilateral or bilateral and located anywhere about the head or neck. Forty percent of headaches are bilateral; 60% are unilateral. It may be mild or severe, with a throbbing, pulsating quality, though these characteristic features are not always present.

The headache may last hours to days but rarely less than 4 hours in duration. Some attacks can last weeks. Severe, debilitating, prolonged attacks are referred to as *status migrainosis* or *intractable migraine*.

A small percentage of migraine attacks occur without head pain. Examples include childhood migraine with *"migraine equivalents"* only, and in the adult, *late onset migraine (transient migraine accompaniments)*. Other adult forms unassociated with headache also occur. The diagnosis is established by the presence of typical features and by ruling

TABLE 7.4. **SELECTED FEATURES OF THE AURA**

Visual	Motor	Sensory	Brainstem Disturbances
Scotomata (formed or unformed figures[a]	Hemiparesis Aphasia (See brainstem disturbances)	Hypersensitivity to feel and touch Paresthesiae	Ataxia Loss or change in level of consciousness
Fortification scotomata[a] (zigzag or scintillating figures)		Reduced sensation (hypesthesia) (See brainstem disturbances)	Diplopia Tinnitus or hearing loss Vertigo
Light sensitivity Photopsia (unformed flashes of light)			Dysarthria (See sensory and motor)
Distortions in shape and size			

[a]In "retinal migraine," these occur unilaterally rather than bilaterally.

out other paroxysmal conditions, such as seizure disorder, TIA, pheochromocytoma, etc.

Table 7.5 lists many of the symptoms that can accompany the pain. They overlap the symptoms of the aura. In fact, any neurological, constitutional, autonomic, or emotional symptom may occur as part of the aura or as an accompanying symptom to the headache.

D. The Postdrome

Following a severe attack of migraine, patients often feel tired, "washed out," irritable, and listless, with impaired concentration and general fatigue. Muscle weakness and aching, anorexia or food craving are common. A feeling of euphoria or hypomania may follow or precede the attack.

III. Variant Forms of Migraine
A. Late-Life Migraine

Late-life migraine, also called *transient migraine accompaniments*, described by Fisher in 1980, represents attacks of episodic neurological events after the age of 45, occurring in the absence of headache, and believed to result from migraine pathophysiology. The attacks last up to 72 hours and are frequently characterized by scintillating scotoma, with migrating episodic neurological symptoms, including paresthesiae, aphasia, and other sensory and motor symptoms.

Patients may or may not have previously experienced migraine. The diagnosis can be established only after ischemic vascular disease and other organic causes of episodic neurological symptoms have been ruled out.

TABLE 7.5. **SELECTED FEATURES ACCOMPANYING THE HEADACHE OF MIGRAINE**

Gastrointestinal	*Brainstem features*
Anorexia	Vertigo
Nausea and vomiting	Ataxia
Diarrhea	Loss of consciousness
Visual disturbances	Diplopia
Blurring	Other
Light sensitivity (photophobia)	*Fluid retention/polyuria*
Other	*Autonomic disturbances*
Fatigue/depression/irritability/anger	Hypertension
Mental dullness/hypomania/confusion	Hypotension
Motor abnormalities	Tachycardia/bradycardia
Sensory abnormalities	Nasal congestion
Dysesthesiae/hyperesthesiae	Peripheral vasoconstriction
Phonophobia/hyperacusis	
Pain throughout the body	

B. Basilar (Brainstem) Migraine

Basilar migraine, also called *basilar artery migraine, vertebrobasilar migraine*, or the *Bickerstaff syndrome*, was first linked to a spasm of the basilar artery, but that is no longer considered likely. The condition frequently affects young people, and belongs to the subgroup *migraine with aura*.

The aura reflects involvement of the basilar or brainstem region, and symptoms include:

- Visual field disturbances;
- Dizziness/vertigo;
- Diplopia;
- Ataxia;
- Dysarthria;
- Tinnitus/hearing loss;
- Bilateral sensory and motor disturbances; and
- Changes in the level of consciousness, including loss of consciousness.

A form of *basilar migraine* is called *stuporous migraine* or *confusional migraine*. Symptoms include the subacute onset of stupor, confusion, and/or severe tiredness, often in association with imbalance and other brainstem signs. Obscene utterances and obstreperous behavior are also noted. The EEG is frequently markedly slowed, which can be a striking feature. The condition is often diagnosed erroneously as "hysterical" or due to drug-induced states. Spontaneous improvement occurs in days to a week.

C. Ophthalmoplegic Migraine

This variant of migraine is characterized by repeated acute attacks of headache, associated with diplopia due to paresis of one or more extraocular muscles and often associated with a dilated pupil. Other cranial nerves may be involved. Diagnostic considerations include:

- Diabetic cranial neuropathy;
- Intracranial aneurysm/tumor;
- Tolosa-Hunt syndrome (painful ophthalmoplegia);
- Acute glaucoma;
- Ocular pseudotumor; and
- CNS infiltrative or infectious disease.

D. Hemiplegic Migraine

Hemiplegic migraine occurs in both sporadic and familial forms. It begins in childhood, sometimes as early as 1–2 years, and generally ceases in later life. The hemiplegia, usually part of the aura, may last an hour or longer. Headache follows the hemiplegia or may occur with it. A male predominance appears to exist. CSF pleocytosis may be present.

E. Retinal Migraine

Retinal migraine is characterized by repeated attacks of headache, preceded or accompanied by visual impairment or blindness involving one eye. The visual impairment lasts less than 1 hour. Headache usually follows the attacks but can be simultaneous or absent. Ischemic, embolic disease and other organic causes must be ruled out. Carotid ultrasound studies and CT scan/MRI are recommended.

F. Progressive Migraine (Transformational Migraine)

Progressive migraine, also referred to as *pernicious migraine* and *transformational migraine*, is considered by the authors of this book as a variant of migraine. It will be covered in detail in Chapter 9.

G. Carotidynia

Carotidynia is sometimes described as a variant of migraine. See Chapter 13.

H. Icepick Pain

Icepick-like, jabbing head pain is frequently encountered in migraine patients, occurring during and independent of actual migraine attacks. The phenomenon is also seen in exertional headache syndromes, such as *hemicrania continua* (see Chapter 14). The brief, painful paroxysms are not serious but are often frightening. The pain may occur in the temple, face, or external ear. The mechanism is not understood. Indomethacin and perhaps other NSAIDs may be specifically helpful.

I. Exertional Migraine (See Chapter 14)

IV. Migraine in Childhood

Between 39 and 70% of children experience at least occasional headache. Some authors believe that most childhood headaches are forms of migraine.

Migraine in children is most often similar to adult migraine. GI complaints, mental changes, and abdominal discomfort are more common in children and may be characteristic features of the childhood attacks.

In children, episodic symptoms of disequilibrium, anxiety, nausea and vomiting, nystagmus, or other symptoms can occur in the absence of headache. These symptoms may represent precursors to more typical migraine attacks in later years. The symptoms are sometimes referred to as *migraine equivalents*, and include:

- Dizziness/vertigo/disequilibrium;
- Nausea and vomiting/abdominal pain;
- Sudden irritability;
- Anorexia;
- Sensitivity to light and sound;
- Cyclic vomiting;
- Diarrhea;
- Personality change; and
- Periodic attacks of limb and joint pain.

Children with migraine are often treated effectively with biofeedback and behavioral, cognitive therapies. Medicines should be avoided if possible, but pharmacotherapy, if appropriate, should not be withheld. See Chapter 9 for a more complete discussion of biofeedback application. Dietary restrictions can also be very useful in children (see Chapter 2).

V. Migraine Infarction

Patients with *migraine with aura* may experience neurological deficits lasting 3 or more weeks and associated with CT scan abnormalities. Though this condition is rare, it nonetheless occurs. Its exact nature in relationship to migraine is not known. Oral contraceptives, smoking, and other risk factors which may be important should be controlled when possible in patients with moderate to severe migraine with aura, particularly if symptoms other than visual aura are present.

VI. Migraine and Epilepsy

Migraine and epilepsy can coexist. Both illnesses may share common EEG patterns, including posterior slowing and episodic, paroxysmal features. A pathophysiological association between these two conditions has not been established with certainty. Some seizure patients experience migraine-like headaches before (aura to seizure), during, or following the seizure. Some patients with severe migraine experience loss of consciousness similar to that seen in certain forms of epilepsy.

Moreover, the aura for epilepsy and that of migraine may be similar or in some cases the same, leading to a seizure on one occasion and to a headache attack on another. Patients with overlapping symptoms or substantially altered EEGs may benefit from the use of both or either antimigraine and antiseizure medications.

VII. Migraine-Provoking Influences

Migraine is an illness in which genetic or acquired factors predispose patients to attacks. A variety of external or internal events appear likely to provoke an attack. *Internalized, cyclic rhythms determined by the chronobiological mechanisms of the hypothalamus may be the key factor determining the specific, temporal vulnerability toward a headache.* During this period, other internal as well as external factors may further lower the migraine threshold.

Table 7.6 lists a number of factors considered likely to induce/provoke a migraine. See also Tables 2.2 and 2.3. Reliability of any of these factors is variable, thus explaining the failure of any one to consistently precipitate an attack.

Certain mental states, food craving, excessive tiredness, light and sound sensitivity (perception of bright light or sound), and food taken during the craving are not "provoking factors," as some people have misinterpreted them to be. Actually, they reflect events of the prodrome or aura. By the time these symptoms occur, the attacks have already started!

Hormonal changes represent one of the more important internal biological factors. The most common predictable time for migraine is around the *menstrual period*. Migraine may also worsen in the first phases of *pregnancy* but improve in the latter

---

TABLE 7.6. **SELECTED POTENTIAL PROVOKING FACTORS OF MIGRAINE**

Stress/anger
Missing meals
Sleep (too much or too little)
Certain foods (see Table 2.3, Chapter 2)
Weather changes
Hormonal changes
  Oral contraceptives
  Menstrual periods
  Pregnancy
Certain medicines
Scintillating, flashing, or bright light
Alcohol
Emotional "letdown"
Exhilaration/anticipation
General metabolic or infectious conditions
Localized cranial disturbances
Smoking/ambient smoke
Strong perfume/odors (paint, cleaning solutions, exhaust fumes, etc.)

two trimesters. Migraine may change its frequency and quality around the time of *menopause*, worsening or improving.

Oral contraceptives frequently, but not necessarily, aggravate migraine. Rarely they relieve migraine. Moreover, the use of *supplemental estrogens* at or around the time of menopause may worsen the attacks. Exceptions are common. The use of synthetic estrogens, such as estradiol (Estrace, Estraderm) or estropipate (Ogen), has anecdotally reduced this aggravating influence, as compared with the use of animal-derived estrogen (Premarin).

VIII. Specific Diagnostic Testing

The neurological examination is usually normal, except in the presence of migraine with aura or complicated migraine. Occasionally, "soft" sensory findings are present.

No clinically available diagnostic test establishes the presence of migraine. *The clinician must exclude other conditions that may mimic or overlap symptoms of migraine, or coexist with it* (see Chapters 2 and 4).

Clinically, provocation by specific instigating factors is a reliable clue. The association of the following factors with migraine gives support for the diagnosis:

1. Headache occurring within minutes to an hour or two after the ingestion of red wine;
2. Headache occurring exclusively at or around the time of a menstrual period;
3. Headache occurring after emotional "letdown";
4. Headache associated with sleeping later than usual; and
5. Headache provoked by weather changes.

The presence of a family history and characteristic clinical features similarly support the diagnosis.

Nonetheless, migraine may be imitated by organic disease (see Chapter 4) and aggravated by coexistent disease. A thorough evaluation is recommended, and may include a CT scan or MRI, EEG, ECG, and metabolic studies to determine the diagnosis or a safety baseline for pharmacotherapy.

IX. Principles of Treatment

As in all headache disorders, the most fundamental principle of treatment is establishing the correct diagnosis. A detailed compilation of information regarding the character of the attacks, provoking and relieving factors, and accompaniments is essential.

In approaching migraine therapeutically, there are two strategies of treatment:

- Treating the individual attack (symptomatic, abortive, reversal therapy); and
- Preventing an attack (prophylactic therapy).

Symptomatic and preventive measures are available in both pharmacological and nonpharmacological forms.

A. Nonmedicinal Therapy

There are relatively few means of symptomatically reversing a migraine attack without medication. Actions that can be taken include:

- Applying ice;
- Taking refuge in a cool, quiet dark environment;
- Practicing biofeedback and relaxation techniques; and
- Inducing sleep.

Avoiding provoking factors and utilizing biofeedback and behavioral and stress management techniques, along with improvement in general health, can be helpful. Biofeedback and cognitive/behavioral treatment can be extremely useful and aid in avoiding medicines in some cases. See Chapter 9 for a more complete discussion of biofeedback and behavioral treatment for headaches.

The following are some additional recommendations:

1. Discontinue smoking;
2. Exercise regularly;
3. Keep day-to-day activities the same, as much as possible; and
4. Avoid foods and circumstances that may provoke headache.

Migraine patients appear somewhat unable to adjust to significant variations from the "norm." Weekend and holiday changes in the patterns of living, for example, make patients quite vulnerable. Attempting to stabilize activities such as eating times and patterns, sleeping (retiring and awakening), stress, and pleasure activities may bring benefit to some patients with headache. Many migraine patients regulate their schedules compulsively as a result of this phenomenon. We refer to this process as *chronobiological stabilization.*

B. The Pharmacotherapy of Migraine

(Details of dose and medication administration can be found in Chapters 5 and 6.)

1. Symptomatic vs. preventive approaches

Both a symptomatic and a preventive approach can be used. Employing each approach simultaneously is required when attack frequency warrants preventive measures and breakthrough headaches require symptomatic treatment. Even under the best preventive circumstances, acute attacks may occur.

a. *Symptomatic therapy*—To reverse or control the headache and accompaniments once the attack has begun.

b. *Preventive therapy*—To minimize the frequency and intensity of expected attacks.

2. Criteria for symptomatic treatment alone

a. When acute attacks occur no more than two times per week.

b. When use of the symptomatic treatment is effective and not contraindicated by other health factors.

The headache frequency may fulfill the criteria for preventive measures, but certain patients do very well with symptomatic treatments alone and do not exceed safety guidelines for their use.

3. Criteria for preventive treatment

a. When attacks of migraine occur at a frequency greater than two attacks per week.*

b. When despite the infrequency of attacks, the devastating nature of the condition makes the use of daily (preventive) medication clinically justified.

c. When symptomatic medications are contraindicated or ineffective.

4. Principles of treatment

a. Provide sufficient but not excessive symptomatic treatment, perhaps with alternatives for moderate and severe attacks, with firm limits on frequency and usage per week.

b. Use rectal or parenteral forms of medication when attacks are accompanied by significant nausea or vomiting or when there is evidence of delayed GI absorp-

---

Many patients with four to eight attacks per month do well with symptomatic treatment alone. Individual consideration is essential. Alternately, menstrual migraine, occurring once per month, may require preventive treatment only at or around the time of menses (see later).

tion (gastroparesis) (often present in even mild to moderate headache attacks).

   c. Adjunctive oral metoclopramide can be used to reverse gastroparesis and improve absorption from the GI tract when oral symptomatic drugs are administered.

   d. Administer rectal or parenteral forms of symptomatic medication (ergotamine suppositories, indomethacin suppositories, parenteral DHE, ketorolac, etc.) for attacks that are not responsive to oral medication.

   e. Employ preventive treatment when criteria are met; provide symptomatic treatment for breakthrough attacks.

   f. Develop a program of symptomatic and preventive medication, sometimes in combination, to establish the most beneficial treatment.

   g. Administer preventive medication for several months, if effective, and then reconsider alternate treatment or impose a "drug holiday."

   h. Provide patients with a range of treatment options for breakthrough attacks. Encourage the avoidance of emergency department treatment except when all means of "at home" therapy have proven ineffective. *Do not deny patients the use of emergency department treatment for acute, resistant headache. In cases of recurring or inappropriate emergency service utilization, consider hospitalization* (see Chapter 6).

   i. Patients with severe attacks who overuse treatment or whose treatments are clearly ineffective should be considered for hospitalization treatment prior to the development of complications and/or addiction/dependency syndromes.

   j. Clinician availability for advice for acute attacks not responsive to "at home" treatment is an essential component of patient compliance and an effective therapeutic relationship.

X. Specific Treatment Approaches
A. Symptomatic Treatment
1. The aura

The aura rarely requires treatment, and it is uncertain whether medications provide any meaningful benefit. The anecdotal use of sublingual nifedipine (10 mg) to reverse focal neurological disturbances has been recommended but is generally unnecessary, since the symptoms usually reverse within 10–20 minutes spontaneously. For particularly severe, recurrent neurologically dramatic aura, nifedipine may be advisable. However, it often worsens the subsequent headache.

2. The headache

For treatment of the headache, the following groups of medications are useful for the acute attack. The reader should refer to Chapters 5 and 6 for tables and descriptions of each of these medications and the method of administration, side effects, and contraindications.

a. Mild to moderate attacks
 1) Simple analgesics, mixed analgesics, hydroxyzine
 2) Nonsteroidal anti-inflammatory agents
 3) Oral antimigraine medications (ergotamine, isometheptene, sumatriptan, if and when available)
b. Moderate to severe attacks
 1) Rectal NSAIDs (indomethacin)
 2) Mixed analgesics (Fiorinal, Esgic, etc.)
 3) Specific antimigraine medications (rectal ergotamine, sumatriptan, if and when available, isometheptene, etc.)
 4) Mixed analgesic/narcotic preparations (containing codeine, oxycodone, hydrocodone, etc.)
c. Severe attacks
 1) Rectal ergotamine
 2) Parenteral DHE (IV, IM, SC)
 3) Parenteral sumatriptan, if and when available
 4) IM ketorolac
 5) Rectal barbiturate
 6) Rectal narcotic (morphine sulfate)
 7) Rectal/parenteral neuroleptic
d. Treatment of nausea, vomiting, and diarrhea
 1) Rectal/parenteral neuroleptics
 2) Oral antidiarrheic agents

B. Preventive Medications for Migraine

1. Categories of medication

The following categories of medication are useful in the prevention of migraine:

a. β-adrenergic blockers
b. Calcium channel blockers
c. Antidepressants (TCA, fluoxetine, MAOI)

    d. Ergot derivatives (methysergide, methylergonovine, ergonovine maleate)

    e. Nonsteroidal anti-inflammatory drugs

    f. Anticonvulsants (valproate, phenytoin, clonazepam, carbamazepine)

2. Principles of preventive medication use

    a. Select appropriate initial agent

    b. Increase dose at a reasonable pace, carefully monitoring for adverse effects, blood pressure, pulse rate, etc.

    c. If treatment is ineffective after several weeks or months at therapeutic levels, add a complementary treatment or discontinue and begin another preventive

    d. Combined preventive treatment is necessary in some difficult-to-control conditions

3. Combination preventive treatment

Combinations of medication may be used for difficult-to-manage cases when risk considerations allow combined usage. Careful monitoring and screening for cardiac, liver, and renal abnormalities, and blood pressure and pulse abnormalities are mandatory. Be aware of additive effects, such as anticholinergic influence (constipation, urine retention, cardiac effects), vasoconstriction, liver toxicity, etc.

Suggested combinations include:

- β-adrenergic blocker and antidepressant;
- Calcium channel antagonist and antidepressant;
- Calcium channel antagonist and ergot derivatives (methysergide, methylergonovine);
- Nonsteroidal anti-inflammatory agent with calcium channel antagonist or β-adrenergic blocker or compatible antidepressant;
- Calcium channel antagonist and anticonvulsant, i.e., valproic acid; and
- MAOI and appropriate TCA (see special instructions, Chapter 5).

Combination treatment should be used with careful and regular monitoring techniques, including regular office visits and metabolic testing.

C. Rebound or Toxic Headache Syndromes

The excessive use of symptomatic medications, including analgesics, ergot derivatives, and perhaps high-dose nonsteroidal anti-inflammatory drugs, can result in a headache/ medication cycle referred to as *rebound headache* or "analgesic rebound headache." (See Chapters 5 and 6)

The *rebound syndrome* is a self-sustaining clinical phenomenon, rendering preventive medications ineffective until discontinuance and withdrawal occur. Withdrawal may require hospitalization and time to stabilize physiological systems until preventive medication can reduce the frequency of attacks, and alternate forms of symptomatic treatment, at restricted intervals, can be employed.

The key features of this syndrome include:

• Insidious increase of headache frequency;
• Dependable and irresistible use of increasing amounts of offending agents at regular, predictable intervals;
• Failure of alternate medications or preventive medications to control headache attacks;
• Development of psychological and/or physiological dependency;
• Predictable onset of headache within hours to days following the last dose of symptomatic treatment;
• Awakening with a headache at the same time each day when this has not been a feature of past headache patterns.

Effective termination of *rebound* can in itself reduce the frequency of headaches. If attempts to reduce the medications result in severe intensification of pain and accompaniments, hospitalization is required (see Chapter 6).

D. Guidelines for Menstrual Migraine

Patients with menstrual migraine often require aggressive and innovative treatments, combining preventive and symptomatic approaches. The following considerations are recommended.

1. Symptomatic treatment

    a. NSAIDs
    b. Ergotamine tartrate (rectal)
    c. Parenteral DHE (self-administered, if possible)
    d. Parenteral sumatriptan (if and when available)
    e. Opiate or related analgesics (oral, rectal, or nasal spray)

2. Preventive treatment

    a. Standard preventive agents, including NSAIDs and ergot derivatives (methylergonovine, methysergide)
    b. Preventive ergotamine tartrate, e.g., daily Cafergot for 4–5 days. (Usage throughout the remainder of the month should be restricted.)

c. Hormonal manipulation (i.e., estrogen patch applied prior to headache onset) (see Silberstein, 1991)

Often, a combined preventive/symptomatic program is necessary. Preventive treatment can be started several days before predictable onset of headache vulnerability and discontinued 2–4 days after menses begins. Menstrual migraine is believed to result from the premenstrual drop of estrogen.

E. Severe Dietary Limitations

A very small percentage of patients with migraine headaches may benefit from severe dietary limitation. Implementation of an elimination diet has been recommended for some of these cases, with good results anecdotally, at least temporarily. Seek dietary consultant for implementation.

8

Tension-Type Headache

I. Introduction

The authors of this book believe that what has been traditionally termed *tension headache* is a form (variant) of migraine. This is a controversial point. Both conditions may be associated with bilateral pain and accompanied by the same clinical features, such as nausea, vomiting, and photosensitivity; aggravated and provoked by many of the same stimuli; have the same male to female ratio and hereditary pattern; and are treated effectively by many of the same medications.

Moreover, epidemiological studies have failed to identify features that could distinguish "tension headache" from migraine on clinical or physiological grounds. The inability to differentiate these two headache types clearly on clinical, epidemiological, therapeutic, and diagnostic grounds has led authorities to believe that indeed they may reflect the same pathophysiological disturbance and should not be considered separately. They may simply represent opposite poles on a broad clinical continuum with migraine at one end and tension or tension-like headache (see Chapter 9) at the other (Raskin, 1988).

After considerable debate and controversy, the International Headache Society's classification employed the term *tension-type headache* for what was previously called *tension headache, muscle contraction headache, stress headache*, and *ordinary headache* (see Table 8.1.)

II. Symptom Overview

The pain of *tension-type headache* is bilateral, dull and aching, and sometimes band-like. The episodic form may last hours to days; the chronic form is persistent and may be continuous.

Patients who earlier in their lives experienced intermittent, typical migraine may evolve to a more frequent, daily or almost daily type of headache, fitting the traditional criteria for "tension headache." Superimposed periodic, acute attacks of migraine accompany the persistent pain. This phenomenon, called *transformational migraine* or *progressive migraine*, may represent one of the most common and difficult-to-treat headache disorders encountered by clinicians. (See Chapters 7 and 9.)

Because we believe that eventually this condition will be defined as a form of migraine and is most effectively treated as though it were migraine, we will not consider this phenomenon further. The reader is referred to the chapter on Migraine (Chapter 7) and the next chapter on Daily Chronic Headache (Chapter 9) for additional perspectives.

TABLE 8.1. **NEW INTERNATIONAL HEADACHE SOCIETY DEFINITION OF TENSION-TYPE HEADACHE**[a]

2.1 *Episodic tension-type headache*
Previously used terms: tension headache, muscle contraction headache, psychomyogenic headache, stress headache, ordinary headache, essential headache, idiopathic headache, and psychogenic headache
Diagnostic criteria:
A. At least 10 previous headache episodes fulfilling criteria B–D listed below. Number of days with such headache <180/year (<15/month)
B. Headache lasting from 30 minutes to 7 days
C. At least two of the following pain characteristics:
    1. Pressing/tightening (non-pulsating) quality
    2. Mild or moderate intensity (may inhibit, but does not prohibit activities)
    3. Bilateral location
    4. No aggravation by walking stairs or similar routine physical activity
D. Both of the following:
    1. No nausea or vomiting (anorexia may occur)
    2. Photophobia and phonophobia are absent, or one but not the other is present
E. At least one of the following:
    1. History, physical, and neurological examinations do not suggest one of the disorders listed in group 5–11
    2. History and/or physical and/or neurological examinations do suggest such disorder, but it is ruled out by appropriate investigations

    3. Such disorder is present, but tension-type headache does not occur for the first time in close temporal relation to the disorder
2.1.1 *Episodic tension-type headache associated with disorder of pericranial muscles*
Previously used terms: muscle contraction headache
Diagnostic criteria:
A. Fulfills criteria for 2.1
B. At least one of the following:
    1. Increased tenderness of pericranial muscles demonstrated by manual palpation of pressure algometer
    2. Increased EMG level of pericranial muscles at rest or during physiological tests
2.1.2 *Episodic tension-type headache unassociated with disorder of pericranial muscles*
Previously used terms: idiopathic headache essential headache, psychogenic headache
Diagnostic criteria:
A. Fulfills criteria for 2.1
B. No increased tenderness of pericranial muscles, if studied, EMG of pericranial muscles shows normal levels of activity
2.2 *Chronic tension-type headache*
Previously used terms: chronic daily headache
Diagnostic criteria:
A. Average headache frequency 15 days/months (180 days/year) for 6 months fulfilling criteria B–D

TABLE 8.1. **CONTINUED**

B. At least two of the following pain characteristics:
   1. Pressing/tightening quality
   2. Mild or moderate severity (may inhibit but does not prohibit activities)
   3. Bilateral location
   4. No aggravation by walking stairs or similar routine physical activity
C. Both of the following:
   1. No vomiting
   2. No more than one of the following: Nausea, photophobia, or phonophobia

D. At least one of the following:
   1. History, physical, and neurological examinations do not suggest one of the disorders listed in groups 5–11
   2. History and/or physical and/or neurological examinations do suggest such disorder, but it is ruled out by appropriate investigations
   3. Such disorder is present, but tension-type headache does not occur for the first time in close temporal relation to the disorder

2.2.1 *Chronic tension-type headache associated with disorder of pericranial muscles*
2.2.2 *Chronic tension-type headache unassociated with disorder of pericranial muscles*

"From Headache Classification Committee of the International Headache Society. Classification and diagnostic criteria for headache disorders, cranial neuralgias, and facial pain. Cephalalgia 1988;8 (Suppl 7): 1–96.

9

Daily Chronic Headache

I. Introduction

For practical reasons, this chapter will discuss those headaches that occur in a daily or almost daily pattern *and* which the authors believe reflect the clinical manifestations and variations of migraine. Some cases of daily chronic headache will have progressed or transformed from patterns of periodic, acute migraine events. Others will begin their headache years with this persistent pattern (new-onset daily headache).

Admittedly, the term *daily chronic headache* is seriously inadequate. Taken literally, the term would include *any* headache, from whatever origin, that occurs daily or almost daily. Thus, it could be used to describe *organic* headache disorders, as well as a variety of other headache syndromes producing daily head, neck, or face pain.

In this chapter, however, the term refers to variations of migraine. The organic causes of headache that could produce a daily pattern will be considered in separate chapters, as will post-traumatic headaches.

The concept of daily chronic headache will include:

* Transformational migraine (progressive migraine, pernicious migraine, etc.), with and without rebound (see below);
* New-onset, daily, persistent headache (onset of daily headache without a transformational component or evolution from episodic migraine pattern); and
* Chronic tension-type headache.

II. Key Clinical Features

Typically, patients with daily chronic headache, as defined here, will experience daily or almost daily, mild to moderate pain, usually bilaterally, and frequently accompanied by neck pain. Periodically, acute attacks of migraine will occur, ranging from four to five attacks per week to monthly or less often.

As is the case with more traditionally defined migraine, a female predominance is present.

A. Transformational Migraine (progressive migraine, etc.)

Transformational migraine specifically refers to the presence of periodic, acute migraine that over time "transforms" or progresses to a more frequent and then continuous pattern, with superimposed acute attacks. The syndrome frequently, but not always, occurs in the presence of increasing use of symptomatic medication ("rebound headache"), which may incite the transformation in some, but not all, instances. Overuse of analgesics or ergotamine tartrate may be a *consequence* rather than a provoking influence.

The transformation of migraine may reflect a variety of other factors, including genetic, psychological, internal or external physiological events (i.e., hormonal), traumatic mechanisms, among others.

B. Clinical Features of Transformational Migraine

Table 9.1 lists the clinical features of transformational migraine.

III. Diagnostic Studies

There are no diagnostic studies to establish the diagnosis of daily chronic headache as a form of migraine. Because of the daily pattern, however, it is essential to rule out head and neck organic pathology, including intracranial obstructive disease, dental disease, CNS ischemia, vasculitis, intracranial infection, systemic disease, and others (see Chapters 4 and 11).

IV. Principles of Treatment

Table 9.2 identifies the principles of treatment of daily chronic headache.

V. Specifics of Treatment

A. Nonmedical Treatment

Nonmedical treatment, including biofeedback, stress management, cognitive therapy, family therapy, substance overuse counseling, life-style changes, exercise, and other health-related adjustments, is important and perhaps essential. (For further discussion, see items D and E.)

TABLE 9.1. **CLINICAL FEATURES OF TRANSFORMATIONAL MIGRAINE**

Intermittent migraine by age 20–30 years
Between ages 25 and 40, gradual increase in headache frequency
Daily or almost daily mild to moderate head, neck, or face pain
Periodic acute severe attacks of migraine, at varying frequency
Frequently occurring accompaniments:
  • Sleep disturbance
  • Overuse of analgesics or ergotamine tartrate
  • Anxiety/depressive states
  • Reduction of quality of life and activities of daily living
  • A family history of headaches
  • A family history of substance overuse, anxiety, or depressive states

TABLE 9.2. **PRINCIPLES OF TREATMENT OF DAILY CHRONIC HEADACHE (PROGRESSIVE MIGRAINE)**

Proper diagnosis (rule out structural, organic disease and treat accordingly, if found)

Reduction of aggravating factors

Reduction of analgesic or ergotamine overuse, if present

Implementation of nonpharmacological treatment (see below)

Implementation of pharmacotherapy (preventive and symptomatic)

Treatment of neuropsychiatric symptoms, such as depression, anxiety, etc.

Assessment of life-style changes, family dynamics, and other factors that might have occurred as a consequence or coexist, aggravating the condition or inhibiting improvement

Education of patients and family regarding the chronic nature of this entity, establishing reasonable expectations and limitations

B. Pharmacotherapy
1. Symptomatic treatment

The treatment of daily chronic headache as a migraine variant consists of the use of symptomatic medications for episodic migraine attacks and preventive therapy for persistent headache. (See Chapters 5 and 6)

2. Preventive treatment

a. Antidepressants. Amitriptyline (Elavil, Endep) and nortriptyline (Pamelor, Aventyl) are currently the most widely used TCAs. Fluoxetine (Prozac) is gaining increasing popularity in the treatment of this disorder but is not yet established as a first-line agent. MAO inhibitors and combinations of medications may be required.

b. β-adrenergic blockers

c. Calcium channel antagonists

d. Ergot derivatives (methysergide, methylergonovine)

e. Anticonvulsants (particularly valproate)

C. Hospitalization

See Chapter 6 for a description of hospital management of headache. Because of the daily presence of interruptive pain, acute episodic attacks, and the frequently associated analgesic or ergotamine overuse patterns, hospitalization to address all factors simultaneously may be necessary. Patients are often unwilling or unable to discontinue analgesics in an outpatient setting because of the escalation of pain that predictably follows, and otherwise acceptable treatments are generally ineffective until analgesics and ergotamine are discontinued and a period of physiological readjustment is established. Substance overuse behavior and other aggravating influences such as disturbed family dynamics make the simultaneous confrontation of these problems essential for effective management.

D. Medication Overuse

Medication overuse is widespread in the headache population, but this often reflects the absence of adequate, more appropriate therapy and should not be interpreted in and of itself as indicative of a primary addictive disorder.

Many experts believe that true *addictive disease* is quite rare in the headache population. More likely, patients who have been inadequately treated desperately seek effective self-treatment for relief and control over their pain and functional limitations. Many could not perform their duties without these medications, and the overuse may be an adaptive effort to maintain some semblance of normal existence. Physical and psychological dependence can occur.

Personality and *borderline character disorders* and true and primary addictive disease are present in some patients with headache. The wise clinician must distinguish between these cases and patients with *inadequately* treated headaches whose use of one or more medication has been prompted by a desperate need to control pain in a medical environment that has failed to address the disorder satisfactorily. These patients are "victims" of the headache disorder and should be seen in this perspective.

E. Psychotherapy, Biofeedback, Cognitive, and Behavioral Treatments

If nothing else, patients with pain need support, understanding, and sometimes expressive therapy.

Nonetheless, within the population of headache sufferers there are those with clearly evident psychiatric, stressful, and behavioral disturbances that contribute to, occur as a response to, or are psychobiological accompaniments to the primary headache problem. Psychobiological accompaniments may arise from the same or related physiological disturbances that cause the headache.

Whatever their origin, the presence of these psychiatric and behavioral disturbances requires proper evaluation and treatment, and successful therapy of these problems may be key to the outcome of headache control.

Psychotherapy itself is rarely adequate to control headache. It should be undertaken within the framework of a broad, comprehensive therapeutic approach that includes pharmacotherapy for significantly painful attacks. Many patients with severe headaches improve psychologically when proper treatment for headaches is achieved, while others experience an improvement in headaches but not depression, anxiety, and other related phenomena. Rarely, patients with severe headaches benefit from psychotherapy and behavioral treatment alone. More often, a comprehensive approach is required.

Biofeedback, stress management, and behavioral/cognitive therapies can help many patients with headache, including those without psychological problems or evident distress, and provide primary, effective intervention. These therapies also serve as adjunctive interventions in patients with frequent headaches who require medicines. Use of these therapies is recommended whenever appropriate. They should be administered by expert professionals well versed in headache disorders.

10

Cluster Headache

I. Introduction

Cluster headache is a devastating, painful affliction. Unlike migraine and daily chronic headache, the condition primarily affects men. Though each attack is relatively brief ($\frac{1}{2}$–$1\frac{1}{2}$ hours), the pain brings with it fear and panicked behavior in many sufferers.

The term "cluster headache" was originally used to describe the clustering or sequence of bouts of painful attacks that occur from weeks to months at a time and then spontaneously terminate. The headache cycle may return weeks or months later. The interval of quiescence is called the *interim*. It is now recognized that a chronic form of cluster headache exists, in which repeating attacks, without interim, occur for years at a time.

The prevalence of cluster headache is reported to be approximately 0.1–0.3% of the population. The attacks can begin at any age, although the majority occur between the ages of 20 and 40 years. Only occasionally is a family history of cluster headache present.

II. Key Clinical Features

Cluster headache is a periodic (30–90 minutes) attack of severe pain primarily localized to the eye, temple, forehead, or cheek region. Up to 50% of patients may have focal tenderness in the ipsilateral occipitocervical junction.

Cluster headache occurs predominantly in males, compared with the female to male ratio (3–4:1) of migraine. The frequency of attacks is 1–6 times per day. Alcohol typically provokes an attack. Statistically, most cluster headache patients are heavy smokers and alcohol drinkers. Attacks frequently occur during sleep or napping times.

Each attack of cluster headache is usually accompanied by ipsilateral lacrimation and nasal drainage, lid drooping, pupillary change, and conjunctival injection.

Table 10.1 lists the clinical features that distinguish cluster from migraine headache.

In *episodic (classic) cluster headache*, the bouts of headache last 1–4 months, followed by an interim. In *chronic cluster headache*, in which an interim does not occur, bouts of head-

TABLE 10.1. **CLINICAL FEATURES DISTINGUISHING BETWEEN CLUSTER AND MIGRAINE HEADACHES**[a]

Feature	Cluster	Migraine
Location of pain	Always unilateral, periorbital	Unilateral, bilateral
Age at onset	Onset in middle age	10–30 years
Sex incidence	Majority male	Majority female
Occurrence of attacks	Multiple daily attacks for several weeks	Usually 2–5 times per month
Time of day	Frequently at night, often same time each day	Any time
Number of attacks	1–6 per day	1–10 per month
Duration of pain	30–90 min	4–24 hours
Prodromes	None	Often present
Nausea and vomiting	2–5%	85%
Blurring of vision	Infrequent	Frequent
Lacrimation	Frequent	Infrequent
Nasal congestion	70%	Uncommon
Ptosis	30%	1–2%
Polyuria	2%	40%
Family history of vascular headaches	7%	90%
Miosis	50%	Absent
Behavior during attack	Paces, pounds fist	Rests in quiet, dark room

[a] Modified from Diamond S, Dalessio DG. *The Practicing Physician's Approach to Headache*. Fifth edition. Baltimore, Williams & Wilkins, 1992.

ache occur for years before termination or remission. The *chronic* form may evolve from the *episodic* form or may have a chronic pattern from its onset.

During an attack, patients will characteristically pace, cry, scream, or pound their fists.

III. Proposed Mechanism

Currently, the exact mechanism of cluster headache remains uncertain.

IV. Specific Diagnostic Tests and Differential Diagnoses

The neurological examination of cluster headache is normal, except for changes during the headache, which might include ptosis, pupillary change, etc. Soft neurological sensory signs may occasionally be present. There are no specific diagnostic tests for cluster headache, although provocation with alcohol is considered a key and reliable feature.

Among the conditions that must be considered are:

• Disease of the orbit;
• Tumors of the brainstem or occipitocervical junction;

- Infiltration/infection of brainstem;
- Cavernous sinus disorders (aneurysm, thrombosis, etc.); and
- Disorders involving the fifth cranial nerve peripheral branches, which may activate central headache mechanisms.
  (See Chapters 4 and 11.)

V. Principles of Treatment
A. Prevention
The primary treatment strategy is *prevention* of the attacks. Symptomatic treatment is adjunctive. Because of the frequency and brevity of attacks, symptomatic treatment is not generally the mainstay of therapy.

B. Regular Medical Visits
Because of the devastating nature of the condition, patients must be seen by their physicians whenever appropriate. Visits cannot be postponed when recurring, untreated attacks are in progress.

C. Aggressive Treatment
Patients must be provided effective and aggressive preventive and symptomatic relief measures. Although steroids (see below) are reliably effective, the risks must be weighed against the benefits. Other preventive agents are often more appropriate first-line treatments.

VI. Specific Treatment Approaches
A. Symptomatic Treatment
Symptomatic treatment includes:
1. Oxygen inhalation*
2. Ergotamine tartrate (rectal, sublingual)
3. Parenteral DHE
4. Parenteral sumatriptan, if and when available

B. Preventive Treatment
The following agents are most appropriate for the prevention of cluster headache:
1. Verapamil is increasingly employed as the treatment of first choice for prevention of cluster headache. It must be administered at relatively high dosages to be effective, 120–160 mg t.i.d.–q.i.d.
2. Steroids are reliably effective (80–90%) in preventing attacks during active therapy. See Chapter 5, Tables 5.11 and 5.12. Though not appropriate for standard preventive therapy, steroids can be used for:
   a. Difficult-to-treat exacerbations

---

*Oxygen (100%) inhalation should be administered via a face mask at 7 liters/min for 10–15 minutes at a time, preferably given at the onset of the attack.

b. At the onset of a cycle to allow time for other medications to take effect

c. As an available "insurance treatment" for breakthrough attacks while traveling or otherwise away from medical care

The risks of steroids must be carefully explained. Continuous steroid treatment should not be used. Repetitive, interval administration should be considered only in truly resistant cases.

3. Lithium
4. Methysergide/methylergonovine/ergonovine maleate
5. Valproate
6. Daily ergotamine tartrate (for otherwise refractory cases)
7. Capsaicin nasal application

VII. Special Considerations

Hospitalization for cluster headache patients may be essential during resistant, severe episodes or when patients become desperate. The use of IV fluids, sedation, parenteral DHE, and other parenteral therapies may be required. Also, patients with cluster headache should avoid alcohol generally, but particularly during cluster cycles. Discontinuing smoking may be very important as well but is quite difficult to achieve. The physician must be very firm on these matters.

A. Cluster Tic Syndrome

The *cluster tic syndrome* features the primary symptoms of cluster headache but with the added component of stabbing, ice-pick neuralgic-like components, involving the eye, face, and jaw. The syndrome is found in 10–20% of patients but is often undiagnosed.

True *trigeminal neuralgia* may coexist with cluster headache.

The treatment is similar to that of cluster headache, with the addition of an antineuralgic program, such as carbamazepine, phenytoin, baclofen, valproate, or clonazepam.

B. Chronic Paroxysmal Hemicrania (CPH)

Chronic paroxysmal hemicrania may be a variant form of cluster headache and is frequently confused with it. A full description is found in Chapter 14.

11

Facial Pain and the Neuralgias

I. Introduction

The diagnosis and treatment of facial pain represents a supreme challenge to the clinician. Facial pain has many causes (see Table 11.1). Historically, pain not clearly identifiable as one of the "typical" (well-delineated) neuralgic syndromes (see later) was assumed to be of psychological origin. Most authorities now, however, believe that many, if not most, facial pain disorders, even if accompanied by depression, arise primarily from physiological dysfunction or organic disease. Psychological issues may represent a comorbid or aggravating condition.

Table 11.1 lists some of the differential possibilities.

II. General Diagnostic Approach
A. Complete History

The history is the key component to a successful evaluation. Factors that must be delineated include:

- Nature of onset;
- Character of pain;
- Location;
- Aggravating and alleviating influences;
- Pattern of pain (constant, periodic, etc.); and
- Other health factors.

Although the location of pain in itself cannot be used to assign origin (pain involving the fifth cranial nerve, other cranial nerves, and cervical spine may be referred to any other region about the head and neck), its location and the presence of tenderness may provide important clues. Pain arising intracranially can be referred extracranially. The reverse is also true. *Pain arising in the right thorax or portions of the gastrum, and innervated by the right vagus nerve, can be referred to the right ear and face.*

Provoking phenomena may suggest etiology. Pain following a dental procedure, aggravated by hot or cold substances in the mouth or from chewing, may suggest dental or jaw origin, whereas pain provoked by cold wind to the face suggests *trigeminal neuralgia*. Pain induced by swallowing or taste stimuli may result from *glossopharyngeal neuralgia, superior laryngeal neuralgia*, or *carotidynia*.

Table 11.1. **SELECTED CONDITIONS CAUSING FACE PAIN**

Neurologic
A. Neuralgic syndromes (trigeminal, glossopharyngeal, etc.)
B. Posterior fossa tumors/aneurysm compressing trigeminal nerves, nervous intermedius, glossopharyngeal or vagus nerves
C. Infiltrative intracranial disease (lymphomatous, etc.)
D. Occipital/cervical and posterior fossa conditions, including Arnold Chiari malformation, type I, obstructive hydrocephalus
E. Postendarterectomy syndrome
F. Cerebrovascular ischemic disease (thalamic pain, etc.)
G. Carotid artery dissection/aneurysm
H. Trauma
 I. Neuritis (trigeminal, optic nerve, occulomotor nerve)
J. Herpes zoster (acute and postherpetic syndromes, including encephalitis)
K. See PRIMARY HEADACHE CONDITIONS
L. Gradenigo syndrome (apical petrositis)
M. Raeder paratrigeminal syndrome
N. Anesthesia dolorosa
Primary Headache Conditions
A. Carotidynia
B. Cluster headache
C. Chronic paroxysmal hemicrania
D. Migraine
E. "Icepick" pain
F. Exertional headache syndromes
G. Phantom tooth pain
H. Others
Dental
A. Tooth abscesses
B. Cracked tooth syndrome
C. Postextraction syndromes
  1. Phantom tooth pain
  2. Postsurgical neuroma
  3. Postsurgical microabscesses
  4. Others
Otolaryngological
A. Sinus disease (infection, infiltrative, tumor, etc.) (See Chapter 4 and Druce, 1991)
B. Bone, jaw disease (infection, infiltrative, tumor, etc.)
C. Nasopharyngeal disease, including carcinoma, peritonsillar abscesses
D. Otalgic disease
  1. External otitis, otitis media
  2. Herpes zoster
E. Nasal septal disease, deviation
Jaw and Cranial Abnormalities
A. Styloid process syndromes (elongation, fracture, etc.)
B. Stylomandibular ligament syndrome
C. Primary disorders of the jaw
D. Myofascial syndromes
E. Neck disease
F. Osteoarthritis of cranial bones
G. Trauma
H. Multiple myeloma
 I. Paget's disease

(continued on p. 124)

Table 11.1. **CONTINUED**

Ocular
A. Refraction errors
B. Heterophoria, heterotropia (weakness of muscles of eye movement)
C. Glaucoma (acute)
D. Corneal and conjunctival disease
E. Ischemic ocular disorders
F. Optic neuritis (retrobulbar neuritis)
G. Herpes zoster ophthalmicus
H. Painful ophthalmoplegia (Tolosa-Hunt syndrome)
Neck Disease
A. Vertebral abnormalities
B. Joint arthritis
C. Disc herniation
D. Root syndromes
E. Osteomyelitis
F. Trauma/fracture
G. Neuralgia (occipital)
H. Tumors
 I. Soft tissue disorders
Others
A. Thoracic tumors (esophageal, pulmonary, and gastric disorders can refer pain to face—usually right ear region) via the auricular branch of the vagus nerve

Pain aggravated by alcohol, exertion, sleep, or menses may suggest migraine or a variant, such as carotidynia. Pain provoked by sneezing, coughing, or exertion may suggest intracranial structural disease, including A-V malformation, aneurysm, posterior fossa structural disease, occipitocervical syndromes, increased intracranial pressure, or "exertional migraine."

Pain demonstrating a distinctive, brief, episodic pattern often suggests a neuralgic origin.

B. Diagnostic Testing

The diagnostic evaluation must be comprehensive if the source of pain and the diagnosis are not clear. A careful evaluation of the cervical spine, cranium, cerebral spinal fluid, and of dental, nasal, eye, throat, sinus, and ear structures is necessary. A complete neurological examination is mandatory.

The following diagnostic studies are recommended, when indicated (see also Chapters 2 and 4):
1. Metabolic evaluation:
   • CBC;
   • ESR;
   • Endocrinological parameters (including thyroid and parathyroid measurements); and
   • General chemistry exam.

2. Standard x-ray examinations
3. CT scan/MRI/MR angiogram (MRA) evaluating head, jaw, and neck (soft tissues and bone)
4. A complete dental and jaw evaluation, including selective alveolar blocks, if appropriate
5. A complete otolaryngological and ophthalmological evaluation, including intra-ocular pressure testing for glaucoma and visualization of nasal, ear, and pharyngeal structures
6. Diagnostic blocks, including occipital nerve, zygapophyseal joints and facet regions of the upper cervical spine
7. An evaluation of soft tissues of the neck, including the carotid artery and glands
8. Evoked response testing (brainstem, visual, somatosensory)

III. Clinical Syndromes
A. Trigeminal Neuralgia
1. Introduction

Trigeminal neuralgia is the most well delineated of the formal neuralgic syndromes. Onset of the disorder is usually later in life (sixth and seventh decades) but can occur earlier. Onset may follow a dental procedure. *Multiple sclerosis* may be causative when present in the younger population.

2. Key clinical features

Brief, unilateral paroxysms of electric-like pain are the primary symptomatic feature. The lancinating pain is in the distribution of one or more divisions of the trigeminal nerve. Maximum intensity of pain lasts a second or slightly longer and occurs repetitively. A sustaining deep, dull ache is often present between acute paroxysms. The pain does not cross to the other side but may be bilateral in 3–5% of cases.

The attacks of pain are characteristically "triggered" by one or more often trivial physical maneuvers (brushing teeth, chewing, talking, cold wind to the face, etc.). A "trigger zone" in the relevant division of the fifth cranial nerve is characteristic, but not always present.

Physical and neurological examinations are usually normal. The presence of impaired sensation along the course of the fifth nerve is atypical and should suggest the possibility of structural or demyelinating or compressive lesions involving the trigeminal nerve, among other possibilities.

Periodic remissions are common, but permanent spontaneous remission are rare. The natural history is variable and unpredictable. A remission of 6 months or more occurs in over 50% of patients.

3. Mechanism

Current theory suggests focal demyelination of the trigeminal nerve, often from vascular compression just prior to entry into the pons (Janetta, 1976). Dental pathology appears capable of activating the syndrome. *Multiple sclerosis* can produce a pattern of pain often indistinguishable from *trigeminal neuralgia* and should be considered in younger patients. Intracranial tumors, aneurysms, and infiltrative disease have produced painful paroxysms, at times indistinguishable from that of *trigeminal neuralgia.*

4. Diagnosis

The diagnosis is established by the characteristic clinical features and by ruling out other pathology. Pain in the distribution of the fifth cranial nerve in association with decreased facial sensation can be the result of trigeminal neuropathy, mandibular or cranial malignancy, and intracranial disease, among other considerations. See II., A. and B. and Table 11.1.

5. General treatment

Patients are desperate and frightened. Some will not eat, drink, brush their teeth, or shave out of fear of activating pain. Aggressive treatment is indicated.

6. Specific treatment

a. Medical treatment

Medical treatment is successful in most patients. Among the useful agents are:

1) Carbamazepine—400–1200 mg/day
2) Phenytoin—300–600 mg/day
3) Baclofen—40–80 mg/day
4) Valproic acid—500–2,000 mg/day
5) Clonazepam—2–8 mg/day
6) Pimozide—4–12 mg/day
7) IV phenytoin—250 mg over 5 minutes

Most of these agents are administered in divided dosages, with the dose increased slowly over several days or weeks, to avoid adverse effects.

Drug combinations may be needed. Baclofen, an often overlooked agent, can be effectively combined with carbamazepine or phenytoin. Phenytoin and carbamazepine can be used together, as can other of the agents.

b. Surgical treatment

A variety of surgical procedures have been used for the treatment of trigeminal neuralgia. Vascular compression of the trigeminal root at the root entry zone is present in 80–90% of patients. This is the basis of the Janetta procedure (Janetta, 1976, 1985), in which via an occipital craniotomy, compression of the trigeminal nerve root by the superior cerebellar artery is relieved. Permanent beneficial results are reported in over 80% of patients. A 1% surgical mortality is present, with serious morbidity in 7%.

Other less invasive, but frequently equally effective, surgical procedures are available, including percutaneous glycerol injection, and radiofrequency rhizotomy.

B. Glossopharyngeal Neuralgia (GN)
1. Introduction

GN is less common than trigeminal neuralgia. The pain is in the distribution of the glossopharyngeal and vagus nerves.

2. Key clinical features

The primary symptoms include: paroxysmal, usually unilateral pain in and around the throat, jaw, ear, larynx, or tongue. Radiation from the oral pharynx to the ear is common. The sudden pain paroxysms along the course of the glossopharyngeal and vagal nerves, including auricular branches, last for about 1 minute. Deep, continuing pain may be present between paroxysms. Multiple attacks per day, up to 30–40, are common and may awaken patients from sleep.

Aggravation by coughing, swallowing, cold liquids, chewing, talking, and yawning is characteristic. Stimulation of the external auditory canal and postauricular area may also provoke pain. Neurological exam is normal, but sensory impairment of cranial nerves IX and X is occasionally present.

In approximately 2% of cases, syncope caused by bradycardia or asystole has been noted, and in some cases seizures, presumably from cerebral ischemia, have occurred. (Atropine prevents bradycardia and fainting, suggesting vagal afferent discharge is the mechanism of the syncope.)

3. Mechanism

The usual cause of GN is vascular compression (as in trigeminal neuralgia) Ectopic impulse formation peripherally is likely to result in disinhibition centrally (similar to that in *trigeminal neuralgia*).

4. Diagnosis

The diagnosis is established by history, physical examination, and ruling out other disease. The following conditions are among those associated with GN-like symptoms:

a. Cerebellopontine angle tumor
b. Nasopharyngeal carcinoma
c. Carotid aneurysm
d. Peritonsillar abscess
e. Osteophytic stylohyoid ligament (lateral to glossopharyngeal nerve)

In 90% of patients tested, local anesthetic to the region of the tonsil and pharynx terminates the pain paroxysms and confirms the diagnosis.

MRI of the head and neck, as well as a careful otolaryngological evaluation, are necessary.

Also, see II. A and B.

5. Treatment

a) *Drug treatment*—same as trigeminal neuralgia
b) *Surgical treatment*—Surgical treatment involves intracranial sectioning of the GN nerve and the upper rootlets of the vagus at the jugular foramen.

C. Superior Laryngeal Neuralgia

1. Introduction

Superior laryngeal nerve, a branch of the vagus, innervates the cricothyroid muscle of the larynx which stretches, tenses, and adducts the vocal cord. Paralysis of the nerve causes hoarseness and fatigued voice, with altered pitch. The syndrome occurs mostly in middle-aged men and may also occur following endarterectomy.

2. Key clinical features

Periodic, unilateral submandibular pain radiating through the ear, eye or shoulder, is characteristic and at times indistinguishable clinically from glossopharyngeal neuralgia. Pain may last seconds to minutes and be provoked by swallowing, straining the voice, turning, coughing, sneezing, yawning, or blowing the nose. An irresistible urge to swallow is noted. A trigger point is frequently present just superior and lateral to the thyroid cartilage.

3. Mechanism

The mechanism is uncertain, but presumably is related to injury or compression of the nerve, as in trigeminal neuralgia.

4. Diagnosis

Same as glossopharyngeal neuralgia.

5. Treatment

Drug therapy is the same as that for trigeminal neuralgia. Superior laryngeal nerve blocking and neurectomy are also available.

D. Sphenopalatine neuralgia

This disorder is known by many names, including *vidian neuralgia, greater superficial petrosal neuralgia, Sluder's neuralgia, pterygopalatine neuralgia*, and others. It may be related to what is now regarded as a recurrent form of carotodynia or cluster headache.

Key clinical features include unilateral pain in the face, usually around the nasal area, typically lasting hours to days, attended by congestion and nasal secretion. It may follow ethmoid sinusitis.

E. Geniculate Neuralgia (Nervus Intermedius Neuralgia)

This syndrome is characterized by lancinating pain in the ear presumably resulting from an alteration in the sensory portion of the facial nerve, the *nervus intermedius*. The syndrome is not distinct from glossopharyngeal neuralgia. Accompanying hemifacial spasm and ear pain are occasionally noted.

F. Occipital Neuralgia

1. Introduction

Occipital neuralgia is a neuralgic-like syndrome involving the greater occipital nerve (GON), a continuation of the dorsal ramus of C-2. The GON enters the scalp between the sternocleidomastoid and trapezius muscles. Compression induces paresthesiae or dysesthesiae.

Tenderness of this nerve or region is frequently encountered in patients with headaches (migraine or cluster headache) and without direct apparent involvement of the nerve, except perhaps by referral. The occipital area, but not specifically the nerve, is the site of referral of pain from upper cervical spine and facet joint disturbances.

The majority of pain authorities believe that true *occipital neuralgia* is generally secondary to traumatic injury. It may be injured in some cases of flexion extension injury (whiplash) and other closed head injury syndromes. *Postherpetic neuralgia* may also occur in this area and affect the nerve.

Occipital migraine and other causes of occipital pain (such as those arising from C2-C3 upper cervical regions) may be misdiagnosed as *occipital neuralgia* (see Bovim, 1992a and b; see also Chapter 17).

2. Key clinical features

The primary clinical features include continuous or paroxysmal pain from the occipitocervical junction, radiating anteriorily; reduced sensation and paresthesias or dysesthesias in the affected distribution of the nerve. Local tenderness is common.

Pain may be referred to ipsilateral frontal, vertex, and eye areas, as well as to the occipital and parietal regions of the scalp.

3. Mechanism

The mechanism of pain is likely secondary to traumatic, infectious (zoster), or chronic compressive disease of the greater or lesser occipital nerves. Neuroma development secondary to trauma is possible.

4. Diagnosis

The diagnosis should be considered when typical features are present and temporarily ameliorated by local blockade. However, the syndrome of *occipital neuralgia* may be mimicked by cervicogenic pain arising from the trapezius muscle, referral from atlanto-occipital joint and upper cervical segments, zygapophyseal and facet joints, C2-C3 roots, and migraine or cluster headache.

Moreover, a blocking procedure in this area may relieve the pain of migraine and other referred conditions and therefore should not in itself constitute confirmation of the diagnosis.

A careful evaluation of the upper cervical spine and posterior fossa is mandatory. Myofascial syndromes should be considered when paraspinal muscle and trapezius tenderness is present.

5. General treatment

Repetitive nerve blocking is helpful in many instances. Carbamazepine and indomethacin have also been found to be useful. Neurolysis and neurectomy may be of benefit in selected cases.

G. Atypical Facial Pain (AFP)

1. Introduction

The term *atypical facial pain* generally reflects the presence of continuous, deep, often burning pain in the absence of clear features defining the more delineated facial pain syndromes. The term *facial pain of unknown cause* used by Raskin (Raskin, 1988) is more appropriate. Despite assumptions regarding a psychiatric origin, association with organic or physiological causes is likely, though not always identifiable.

2. Key clinical features

Continuous unilateral (occasionally bilateral) pain or discomfort occurs in the distribution of the cheek, eyes, temples, gums, nose, or jaw. Women are more commonly affected than men. Depression with or without anxiety is a frequent accompaniment. Patients are often frightened, withdrawn, angry, and demoralized from pain as well as from rejection by health care professionals. They are vulnerable to a variety of inappropriate explanations and fad therapies.

3. Diagnosis

See II. A. and B.

The following conditions should be considered and excluded, if appropriate.

a. Maxillary and mandibular bone disease

Pain arising from occult, infected maxillary or mandibular bone cavities from previous tooth extractions is a major undetected cause. Oral surgical evaluation and blocking is required. Local selective alveolar blocks in the site of the tooth extraction is diagnostic. Curettage of the bone with antibiotic treatment is recommended.

b. Phantom tooth pain

Phantom tooth pain is a deafferentation disorder which results in pain in the region of previous tooth extractions. Recent studies by Sicuteri (1991) suggest a high correlation with a history of migraine or cluster headache. The condition responds to standard migraine or cluster headache treatment and perhaps to the neuralgic treatments as well.

c. Post-traumatic facial pain

Trauma to the face often produces chronic facial pain, as can previous surgical trauma. The pain usually is self-limited, often subsiding 1–5 years after onset. The mechanism is presumed to be activation of central pain transmission pathways, but the exact mechanism is yet to be determined.

d. Anesthesia dolorosa

Painful anesthesia is a dysesthetic syndrome following trauma to the trigeminal nerve or other cranial nerve, often following surgical treatment for neuralgia. Its primary symptom is burning pain. The pain is difficult to treat and frequently requires aggressive pharmacological and nonpharmacological intervention. Depression is common. Anticonvulsant, antineuralgic therapies may be of benefit, as are antidepressants.

e. Thalamic pain

Thalamic pain presents as a unilateral facial pain with dysesthesia and usually follows ischemic lesions in the thalamus. Trunk and limb pain is also usually present. The pain is often of sudden onset and occurs most frequently in patients with ischemic disease or multiple sclerosis. Because the syndrome has been identified in patients with lesions in the brainstem, and without apparent involvement of the thalamus, the term central post-stroke pain (CPSP) may be more appropriate (Leijon, 1989).

f. Other causes

The role of psychiatric disease in atypical facial pain is a matter of controversy. Nondescript facial pain can be present and accompanied by significant depression and anxiety, which can also accompany all other forms of chronic pain. The coexistence of depression does not alone suggest a causal relationship and is better explained by the concept of comorbid disease or reactive, desperational phenomena. The absence of identifiable, objective cause should not in and of itself justify or constitute the establishment of psychogenic origin. The absence of objective markers may be better explained by the failure of diagnostic science than the psychiatric profile of the patient. Patients have had medical ailments long before doctors have identified causes or tests to diagnose them.

4. Treatment

Treatment consists of employing varying combinations of the following medications:

a. Antidepressants

b. Antineuralgic agents

c. Migraine drugs

d. Cluster headache drugs

Among the antidepressants, amitriptyline, nortriptyline, phenelzine, and desipramine are particularly valuable.

Atypical facial pain without identifiable cause requires pharmacotherapy. However, patients may benefit from adjunctive and supportive psychological and behavioral therapy.

H. Postherpetic Neuralgia (PHN)

1. Introduction

Postherpetic neuralgia is a neuralgic syndrome resulting from a previous *acute herpes zoster* attack along a specific nerve distribution. It evolves several weeks after the acute attack and is more likely to occur in patients of advanced age.

The acute zoster episode is often preceded by a spectrum of sensory disturbances in the afflicted region, followed 4–5 days later by a vesicular eruption. The most typical areas of involvement in the head and neck are in the distribution of the ophthalmic division of the trigeminal nerve and the occipitocervical junction. Most attacks are unilateral.

Postherpetic neuralgia follows the acute attack of *herpes zoster* by days or weeks and is more likely when the acute attack of zoster is more intense. It is also more common with increasing age, approaching a 50% incidence in the seventh decade and 75% after 70 years of age. It is as low as 5% in patients below the age of 40.

Patients with myeloma have a higher rate of acute infection.

Overall, long-term prognosis is good for *postherpetic neuralgia*, with a spontaneous improvement in pain in the majority of patients. Approximately 5% continue to have resistant pain.

2. Key clinical features

Following the acute eruption, pain may persist or return within weeks to months. Pain usually occurs in areas overlying abnormal skin, which is generally hypesthetic. Hyperesthesia to light touch may also occur. The pain is usually superficial but may have a deep and burning quality. Repetitive stabs of pain and needle pricking sensations are common. Interruption of normal activities, including sleep, is typical. Light touch often provokes paroxysms of discomfort.

Ophthalmic herpes may follow involvement of cranial nerves III, IV, and VI. *Geniculate herpes* is associated with facial palsy (CN VII). Vesicles are apparent in the external auditory canal.

3. Mechanism

It is believed that the initial zoster infection produces inflammatory necrosis of the dorsal root ganglion which may extend to the meninges and dorsal root entry zone of the involved segments. *Postherpetic neuralgia* probably reflects a deafferentation pain syndrome in which sensory nerve injury results in interruption of the involved neuron. The burning pain is often accompanied by increased sympathetic activity.

4. Treatment

a. Treatment for the pain of the *acute zoster* infection:
   1) oral steroids
   2) antiviral agents (acyclovir, vidarabine, and α-interferon)
   3) sympathetic blocks
   That these treatments will actually prevent the development of the postherpetic syndrome has been proposed but not established.

b. Treatment of *postherpetic neuralgia*: The pharmacological treatment for PHN includes combinations of the following:
   1) local application to the affected area of capsaicin cream (0.025% or 0.075%)
   2) amitriptyline up to 150 mg per day
   3) valproate or other antineuralgic agent (alone or in combination with amitriptyline)
   4) perfenazine (a phenothiazine), used in combination with amitriptyline
   5) repetitive intravenous infusions of procaine or lidocaine

c. Surgical treatment: Effective surgical therapy is not available for *postherpetic neuralgia* involving facial regions, but root entry zone lesions have been effective for truncal pain.

I. Temporomandibular Joint Pain (TM Joint Pain)

1. Introduction

TM joint dysfunction and related muscular symptoms (myofacial pain) are poorly defined and poorly delineated syndromes. According to most responsible headache authorities, TM joint dysfunction and related phenomena are overstated and exaggerated as causes of pain and are overtreated, in general. The clinical and basic science related to these disorders is seriously conflicting and rudimentary. Nonetheless, little doubt exists that major disturbances of bite and mandibular function with related muscular disturbances can contribute, if not cause, a variety of painful phenomena. Masticatory muscle spasm and fatigue can produce pain, as can major structural and inflammatory disturbances of the joint.

It is likely that disturbances of jaw and myofascial components aggravate preexisting or latent headache and face pain disorders, such as migraine. Thus, appropriate treatment of the peripheral (jaw and muscular) tissue may help reduce the activation phenomena, if not address the primary source of pain directly. Epidemiological and demographical data on the TM joint and related syndromes are in dispute.

2. Key clinical features

A wide range of painful, unilateral symptoms involving the jaw, face, ear, or preauricular area is noted, with radiation to temple, jaw, and neck. The pain is often deep, persistent, and worsened after clenching, chewing, or wide oral opening. Clicking or "locking" of the jaw is reported by some patients with actual joint abnormalities. Limitation of jaw motion with deviation upon opening is common. Tenderness of the jaw, reduced range of motion, and pain with movement, together with crepitation, are usually present. In myofascial syndromes, muscle tenderness in temporalis and pterygoid muscles is often significant. True jaw dysfunction and/or myofascial symptoms may occur separately or concurrently.

3. Mechanism

The primary mechanism for myofascial pain, according to most responsible authorities, is muscle spasm involving the masticatory muscles leading to malocclusion, bruxism, or teeth clenching. The concept of condylar displacement is controversial and in dispute. The association with rheumatoid arthritis is uncertain. Post-traumatic injuries of the jaw or related soft tissues may be important and overlooked, including mandibular ligamentous or styloid process disruption. These may occur following flexion/extension injury to the neck. Dramatic exacerbation of preexisting jaw pathology also occurs.

4. Diagnosis

See II. A. and B. Of special consideration are:

a. Neuralgic disorders

b. Post-traumatic syndromes, including fracture or elongation of the styloid process

c. Stylomandibular ligamentous syndrome (Ernest syndrome)

d. Referred pain to the ear from vagus branches in the chest, esophagus, or gastrum

Careful physical examination of the jaw, intraoral, auditory, and muscular elements is necessary, as well as an evaluation of the chest (chest x-ray). Vagal branches in the chest, esophagus, and gastrum may be referred to the right aural region.

Physical examination generally reveals four primary findings in true TM joint dysfunction:

1. Pain

2. Tenderness

3. Clicking

4. Limitation of motion

5. Treatment

a. *Conservative therapy* appears to be the most appropriate approach for both myofascial and joint disorders initially. It is effective in most cases. A serious effort at resting and relaxing the jaw and its musculature is mandatory. The methods include:

1) soft diet

2) behavioral/relaxation therapies/biofeedback

3) local heat

4) reduction of gross occlusal disturbances with a bite guard

5) use of NSAIDs

6) jaw exercises

Local injections may be helpful in selected cases.

b. *Surgical procedures* should be avoided, except in extreme circumstances. The results have been inconsistent and can contribute to a worsening spiral of pain, narcotic analgesic overuse, and depression.

6. Additional thoughts

A major problem in the treatment of TM joint dysfunction and related disorders is the frequency with which primary headache conditions represent the underlying primary painful disorder. The TMJ and related conditions should be diagnosed only *after* a full consideration of other etiologies, including serious organic phenomena, have been ruled out (see Bindoff, 1988).

Diagnosis and treatment should occur in the perspective of a broad range of head and face pain syndromes, the predispositional factors which affect people with head and face pain syndromes, and a view that the jaw therapy in itself may be but a component rather than a focus of proper treatment. The use of narcotic analgesics as the mainstay of treatment following surgical intervention may be a serious problem, as can the surgery itself.

Addressing the psychological distress which is often concurrent (comorbid, not necessarily causative) may be equally important.

12

Post-Traumatic Headache and Syndrome
Post-Concussion Syndrome, Post-Traumatic Syndrome

"Though no objective signs accompany these complaints, they are so uniform from case to case that the symptoms cannot be regarded as other than genuine." —H. Cushing, M.D.

I. Introduction

The *post-traumatic syndrome*, also called *post-concussion syndrome* and *subjective post-traumatic syndrome*, is a constellation of symptoms which can follow mild to moderate closed head injury (actual cranial impact). It is also seen following flexion/extension trauma (whiplash) in which no actual cranial contact has occurred. The primary symptoms, usually strikingly consistent from patient to patient, include one or more of the following:

- Headache, neck, and shoulder pain;
- Sleep disturbance;
- Cognitive abnormalities;
- Mood and personality changes; and
- Dizziness, with or without vertigo.

Long a controversial matter, the prevailing view of most authorities is that the condition is a neurological disorder that may arise *even if frank unconsciousness has not occurred.* (Patients with momentary loss of consciousness are often not aware that consciousness was lost and report "NO" to the ER question, "Did you lose consciousness?"). The most appropriate term to describe this condition is *post-traumatic syndrome.* Use of the term "concussion" traditionally implies a loss of consciousness, which is not necessarily present even in bona fide cases of this disorder.

Headache represents the most common symptom in patients with closed head injury, usually persisting for more than 2 months in 60% of patients, even those with apparently minor trauma. The symptoms do not correlate with the presence or duration of unconsciousness, amnesia, or any identifiable neurodiagnostic study. An inverse relationship may exist between the severity of head injury, as determined by the duration of post-traumatic amnesia, and the incidence of headache (Raskin, 1988).

The cynical assumption that protracted cases result from litigation motives or other nonphysiological circumstances is not supported by data. Most experts believe that only a small percentage of patients with protracted syndromes are malingering or embellishing. Rather, studies support the view that enduring and persistent impairment and pain can occur even after minor injury. Moreover, studies do not support the view that impairment is linked to litigational issues (Leininger, 1990, among others).

II. Pathophysiology
A. Neurocognitive and Other Nonpain Symptoms

The exact mechanism for accompaniments is not known but structural changes are seen. Gross and microscopic abnormalities, including brain hemorrhage, occur in animals following carefully controlled head trauma approximating minor head injury in humans. Though few human autopsy reports are available, together with animal studies the following pathology and observations are noted:

1. Nerve cell loss, alteration
2. Vascular disturbances in subcortical, cortical, and brainstem regions
3. Degeneration and damage to microglia and axones
4. That less trauma is required to render unconsciousness if the head is more freely mobile
5. Head rotation during impact may be a critical factor determining injury and sequalae
6. That even in the absence of direct impact, concussion may be produced by rotational displacement

B. Pain Symptoms

The precise mechanism for head pain remains elusive. Patients may experience both extracranial and intracranial injury. Among the proposed pain-producing mechanisms are (see Chapter 17 for further discussion):

1. Extracranial and cervical soft tissue injury (muscle, tendon, blood vessel, nerve)
2. Intracranial disturbance (physiological, microstructural) of brainstem pain-modulating mechanisms
3. Cervical root, spinal cord, facet joint, atlantoaxial vertebra, and TMJ injuries, etc., in addition to other soft

tissue and bony alterations, including those of the sty-lomandibular ligament area

4. Ischemic brainstem and vestibular disturbance, perhaps secondary to vertebral artery spasm

C. Predispositional Conditions

"It's not so much what happens to the head, but whose head it happens to." (Modified from Symonds, 1937)

Neurobiological and neuropsychiatric predispositional factors may explain why some patients subjected to mild to moderate head injury experience one or more of the sequelae, while others do not. Nonetheless, the symptoms seem bona fide in most cases.

III. Key Clinical Features

Both immediately apparent symptoms and delayed phenomena (perhaps not initially recognized or evident) may occur. The delayed symptoms might result from a requisite interval between trauma and pathophysiological manifestation (as in *delayed post-traumatic epilepsy, delayed post-traumatic encephalopathy,* etc.) or reflect features that have not become apparent until convalescence was complete and normal function and high-level cognitive demands were present.

A. Pain and Headache

Headache, neck, and shoulder pain are usually present within the first 24–48 hours, although days or weeks may pass before onset. Neuralgic-like syndromes of the frontal or occipital regions may not appear for months or longer. The pattern of pain may change and the intensity fluctuate over months and years.

Several pain patterns are noted:

1. Generalized, bilateral, persistent mild to moderate headache, similar to daily chronic or tension-type headache
2. Neuralgic-like pain in occipitocervical or frontal regions (see Chapter 11)
3. Periodic, throbbing migraine-like attacks, sometimes accompanied by scintillating scotoma and other migrainous features, including nausea, light sensitivity, etc. May be occipital in location
4. A cluster headache-like syndrome
5. Suboccipital and cervical pain, with and without movement, perhaps from injury to suboccipital muscles, upper cervical vertebrae, zygapophyseal joints, etc.
6. Cervical radiculopathy secondary to root injury

7. Myofascial-like pain with "trigger points" in the occipital, cervical, shoulder (trapezius, supraspinatus), and paraspinal regions
8. A low-pressure headache pattern (with postural aggravation)
9. A brachial plexus-like syndrome (EMG rarely confirmatory) with features of positional arm and shoulder pain and headache aggravation following shoulder and arm exertion
10. TM joint/myofascial syndrome, including injury to the joint itself, styloid process (fracture), styloid ligament, etc.

The majority of patients experience features of one or more of these patterns. Referred phenomena from suboccipital regions to frontal, vertex, or orbital regions have been documented and may account for the frequency of complex pain patterns (see Chapter 17).

B. Neurocognitive Impairment

Impaired memory, minor to major cognitive deficits, and reduced concentration are present in a significant number of patients with *post-traumatic syndrome*. Key features include the inability to process information normally (or at a fast rate) and memory impairment.

C. Neuropsychiatric Phenomena

1. Personality change
2. Depression, with and without anxiety
3. Irritability, with anger outbursts and emotional intolerance
4. Loss of sense of humor
5. Reduced motivation and social interaction
6. Generalized lethargy (mental and physical)
7. Rage attacks
8. Hypomania
9. Hyperkinesis, mood changes, impaired attention, and enuresis (common in children)

D. Vertigo and Dizziness

Frank vertigo, as well as vague, nonspecific dizziness, are common. Positional vertigo may be present in up to 80% of patients reporting dizziness. It is worsened by movement of the head or a rapid change in body position. Imbalance is a common complaint.

E. Sleep Disturbance

Sleep disturbances, including insomnia, frequent nocturnal awakening, and daytime sleepiness, are common.

F. Spells

A variety of seizure-like events is reported in this group. These include:

1. True syncope (occurs rarely)
2. True epilepsy (occurs rarely)
3. A variety of nonspecific periodic, paroxysmal events (pseudoseizures?), including:
   a. Staring spells
   b. Nonvestibular dizziness
   c. Sudden loss of memory (amnesia or confusion)
   d. Narcolepsy/cataplexy-like spells
   e. Episodic disorientation and fugue-like states

The term "pseudoseizure" does not necessarily imply the absence of physiological legitimacy. Though it is broad and may embody nonorganic circumstances, the term is used here to describe what appears to be physiological, bona fide cerebral events which do not fit existing epilepsy criteria.

G. Family Dysfunction

The patient's family also generally suffers as a result of the trauma. Role reversal (dependency by a previously independent family member), rejection, disbelief, and anger toward the injured person are common, contributing to the deterioration of quality and stability of life.

H. Other Symptoms/Signs

1. Weight loss or gain
2. Changes in appetite
3. Increased thirst
4. Alcohol intolerance
5. Menstrual irregularities, including amenorrhea
6. Sexual dysfunction; loss or increase of libido
7. A variety of "soft" neurological findings on examination
8. Others

Traumatic disruption in the area of the hypothalamus and pituitary/adrenal axis is believed to contribute to many of these complaints.

IV. Specific Diagnostic Testing
A. Neurocognitive

The most reliable studies involve neurocognitive evaluation, which often demonstrate impaired neurocognitive function. No other practical, widely available study so consistently demonstrates a basis for many of the features in this condition.

B. Other Recommended Studies and Evaluations, When Appropriate

1. Visual evoked potentials, brainstem auditory evoked potentials
2. Electroencephalography (altered in 10–30% of patients but nonspecific in form)
3. MRI/CT scan of head and neck
4. Special sleep studies, which may demonstrate pattern abnormalities of sleep staging
5. Dental/jaw evaluation
6. Otolaryngological and vestibular evaluation including electronystagmography and other vestibular testing
7. Diagnostic nerve blockade (vertebral, supraorbital, paravertebral and suboccipital regions)
8. Positron emission tomography testing (PET scanning); not yet of practical value but has demonstrated changes that could explain post-traumatic behavioral disturbances (Starkstein, 1990). The test offers promise for future clinical substantiation of this condition.

C. Key Clinical Elements

The key clinical elements to establishing the diagnosis are:

1. The convincing presence of symptoms that are consistent with the key features of the syndrome
2. A comprehensive history of the traumatic event and sequelae, which, when compared with pretraumatic medical status, cognitive function, and job or school performance, supports that a significant change in clinical status and cognitive function has occurred within a compatible temporal relationship to the injury
3. The careful exclusion of other physiological, psychological, or organic disorders that might mimic or coexist with the symptoms of *post-traumatic syndrome*, including:
   a. Subdural/epidural hematoma
   b. CSF hypotension
   c. Cerebral vein thrombosis/cavernous sinus thrombosis, fistula, aneurysm
   d. Cerebral hemorrhage
   e. True seizures
   f. Post-traumatic hydrocephalus
   g. Vertebral/cervical root/suboccipital injury
   h. Jaw, TM joint, styloid ligament or process, facial injury

V. Principles of Treatment

Patients with post-traumatic syndrome are generally seriously distressed and seriously misunderstood. Appropriate treatment requires an objective, approach to the complaints. Most patients are neither embellishing nor malingering. An objective, unbiased (neutral) appraisal is essential. This requires a comprehensive data collection process and a detailed, well-designed diagnostic evaluation. Neurodiagnostic testing and the performance of sufficient other studies to rule out coexistent or mimicking illness may then support the presence of this syndrome by exclusion.

VI. Specific Treatment Approaches

A comprehensive approach to treatment is frequently required.

A. Headache and General Pain

1. Patients should be treated in the manner described in other sections of this book for various headache patterns, if migraine, daily chronic headache, or related syndromes are apparent.
2. Cervical and shoulder syndromes and/or neuralgic-like syndromes may benefit from:
   a. Trigger point injection
   b. Various nerve and joint blocking procedures
   c. Physical medicine therapies, including TNS
   d. Pharmacotherapy, using antidepressants, antineuralgic agents, muscle relaxants, and nonsteroidal anti-inflammatory drugs
3. Biofeedback and relaxation therapy
4. Specific treatment for jaw or neck injury

B. Spells

If true seizure activity is present, appropriate anticonvulsant therapy is indicated. Many patients do not benefit from standard anticonvulsant treatment but may benefit from "stimulant-type" medication. Fluoxetine and other "activating" antidepressants, methylphenidate, and pemoline have been of anecdotal benefit.

C. Neurocognitive Dysfunction

Individually designed cognitive retraining, counseling, and vocational rehabilitation are often necessary. Head injury support groups can be helpful.

D. Family Dysfunction

Family therapy, and consultation with employer and school personnel, is recommended when appropriate. Careful explanation of cause, mechanism, and prognosis is helpful to all involved, particularly the patient.

Many patients with *post-traumatic syndrome* will require aggressive, multifaceted, therapeutic programs involving:
- Physical measures (physical therapy, nerve blocks, TNS, trigger point injections, etc.)
- Pharmacotherapy (antidepressants, β-adrenergic blockers, DHE, etc.)
- Rehabilitative and supportive psychotherapeutic efforts

VII. Special Considerations

The validity of this disorder cannot be proven objectively at this time. Such has been the early history of many "neurobiological illnesses," including autism, Tourette's syndrome, epilepsy, schizophrenia, and chorea, to name but a few. Objective and prudent clinical observation and common sense support the view that traumatic assault to delicate neural circuitry is likely to result in the disturbances that account for the symptoms reported.

In most instances, the absence of objective markers is explained by the absence of sufficient diagnostic sophistication, not the legitimacy of the complaints. As stated earlier, patients have experienced symptoms long before doctors have known how to diagnose or treat them, or even that they exist at all.

Delayed sequelae are possible and familiar to many neurological conditions, including post-traumatic epilepsy. Early recognition of the impairment followed by aggressive, well-designed intervention may help prevent physiological and emotional deterioration.

Key factors in determining prognosis are the attitudes and skills of the physician in charge of care. Objectivity must be maintained, and direct physician involvement in the strategy and delivery of treatment is necessary. Symptoms may persist for years and even a lifetime, despite qualified and appropriate interventions. Knowledgeable physicians must directly influence planning of current and future treatment and anticipated patient needs. These factors are very important not only to patients, but to family and support agencies as well.

In short, this condition can no longer be denied physiological legitamacy with such compelling clinical support for its existence. Cynicism must give way to objective neutrality in the face of strong, albeit subjective, clinical evidence.

13

Carotidynia and Carotid Artery Dissection

Introduction

Syndromes of carotidynia and carotid artery dissection will be considered together, because both represent anterior neck pain syndromes and are assessed in a similar fashion.

I. Carotidynia

A. Introduction

Carotidynia refers to pain arising from the region of the cervical carotid artery, frequently radiating to the jaw, face, ear, and head on the ipsilateral side. Both acute and chronic forms exist. *Carotidynia* is a frequently overlooked cause of recurring facial pain (see Chapter 11). Dental trauma may be an important precipitant.

B. Key Clinical Features

1. Acute carotidynia

The acute or subacute onset of pain (stabbing, throbbing, or dull) lasts days to months (average 12 days). The pain is typically unilateral but bilateral pain has been reported. The syndrome may result from an upper respiratory infection. The pain is aggravated by neck and head motion, swallowing, sneezing, yawning, and coughing.

2. Chronic carotidynia

The chronic form of carotidynia is more well known and was initially identified in patients with chronic facial pain. Most patients are women, and an association with migraine is noted. The carotid artery is tender, and headache may or may not be an accompaniment.

The pain is persistent and is usually located in the neck, jaw, and periorbital regions. Periorbital and maxillary pain are not uncommon. The pain is dull, with throbbing elements. Periodic exacerbation lasting up to hours is noted. Icepick-like jabs are noted (see Chapter 7).

Tenderness and prominent pulsations, along with soft tissue swelling overlying the carotid artery on the ipsilateral side, are characteristic.

C. Mechanism

The primary mechanism of carotidynia may be similar to migraine and may represent a migraine variant (see Chapter 7). Moreover, studies demonstrate that electrical stimulation of the carotid artery wall at its bifurcation can produce pain in a variety of areas about the head and jaw. Denervation of the carotid artery produces cessation of facial pain.

D. Diagnosis

1. The diagnosis is established by ruling out other painful disorders of the neck, including:
   a. Giant cell arteritis
   b. Spontaneous carotid dissection
   c. Carotid atherosclerosis
   d. Thyroiditis
   e. Ruptured cervical carotid artery aneurysm
   f. Fibromuscular dysplasia
   g. Cluster headache/migraine
   h. Elongation/fracture of styloid process
   i. Tumor
2. Recommended studies:
   a. MRI of the neck (MR angiogram of carotids)
   b. CT scan/MRI of head
   c. Ultrasound of carotid artery
   d. Carotid arteriogram (rarely required in carotidynia)
   e. Appropriate blood and metabolic studies

E. Specifics of Treatment

1. The acute syndrome:
   a. Prednisone 60 mg, or
   b. Triamcinolone 24 mg
      Administer for 7 days, followed by gradual reduction (see Tables 5.11, 5.12, Chapter 5)
2. The chronic syndrome is treated with one or more of the following:
   a. Indomethacin 25–50 mg t.i.d.
   b. Methysergide/methylergonovine
   c. Propranolol
   d. Nortriptyline
   e. Other migraine or cluster headache treatment

II. Carotid Artery Dissection

A. Introduction

Acute headache and neckache in the presence of stroke-like neurological symptoms are the primary features of *spontaneous dissection of the internal carotid artery*. The syndrome was first described in 1959 and is sometimes associated with the following phenomena:

1. Migraine
2. Fibromuscular dysplasia
3. Cystic medial necrosis
4. Marfan's syndrome
5. Arteritis
6. Atherosclerosis
7. Other congenital abnormalities of the arterial wall

Dissection of vertebral arteries has also been reported.

B. Key Clinical Features

1. Sudden onset of headache, retro-orbital, or neck pain
2. Acute neurological events
   a. Incomplete Horner's syndrome
   b. Confusion
   c. TIA or ischemic stroke symptoms (from anterior or basilar vascular systems)
   d. Carotid bruit

C. Mechanism

Apparent weakness of the arterial wall, resulting in separation of the internal elastic lamina from the medial layer, is a consistent finding. Extravasation of blood into the arterial wall produces hematoma, with occlusion of the lumen.

D. Diagnosis

The diagnosis of carotid artery dissection requires ruling out other causes for neck and head pain accompanied by neurological symptoms (see I. D.).

Historically, the diagnostic procedure of choice has been arteriography. MRI of the soft tissues of the neck and/or MRI angiography of the carotids, however, may be quite valuable. A well-performed Doppler ultrasound examination may also be helpful.

Because the acute neurological symptoms frequently prompt an aggressive pursuit of intracranial pathology, the vasculature in the neck is often overlooked.

E. Treatment

Anticoagulation and surgical intervention can be considered on a case-by-case basis. No controlled studies are available.

14

Headaches Provoked by Exertional Factors and Responsive to Indomethacin

I. Introduction

Several headache syndromes share the features of being provoked by physical stimulation (exertion, cough, flexion/extension of the neck), and response to indomethacin. Many have a relationship to migraine and may respond to migraine therapy as well (see Chapters 5 and 7).

The exact mechanism of these disorders is not known, but they may result from sudden and/or repeated intracranial pressure elevations (Raskin, 1988).

II. Specific Syndromes

A. Cough Headache/Benign Exertional Headache/ Effort Migraine

1. Introduction

The term *cough headache* refers to an exertional headache syndrome in which severe but transient headache occurs subsequent to a variety of exertional, straining activities, including but not limited to:

a. coughing
b. sneezing
c. straining
d. weightlifting
e. bending
f. stooping

Initially considered an ominous sign, it is now considered likely to be of benign origin, although structural/organic causes must be ruled out. The condition is sometimes named *benign exertional headache, benign cough headache,* or *effort migraine.*

2. Key clinical features

A severe, usually bilateral, sudden-onset headache occurs within moments after an exertional stimulus, subsiding within seconds in the case of cough headache and within 5–24 hours in the benign exertional headache and effort migraine. Dull aching may persist for hours, but between attacks patients are generally pain-free. Patients may be prone to other chronic headaches.

The location is often diffuse but can be lateralized. Accompaniments are generally absent, but effort migraine has been associated with transient neurological events and nausea and vomiting. These are more likely when the syndrome occurs at high elevations and in warm temperatures.

3. Diagnosis

a. Differential diagnosis

Structural/organic causes of exertion or position-induced headache must be ruled out. Among these possible causes are:

1) Intractranial mass lesions (particularly tumors, structural or obstructive abnormalities of posterior fossa or occipital/cervical junction, such as Arnold-Chiari malformation type I)
2) A-V malformation
3) Aneurysm
4) Intracranial hypertension (obstructive, nonobstructive)
5) Cranial sinus (paranasal sinuses, etc.) disease
6) Cerebral venous thrombosis
7) Tumor

b. Testing

1) CT scan/MRI of head. A CT scan with and without contrast is helpful, but an MRI evaluates the presence of structural abnormalities of the posterior fossa and occipitocervical junction more effectively.

The MRI, when done in conjunction with a Valsalva maneuver, is recommended to further assess the presence of tonsillar herniation.

2) An MR angiogram and arteriography must be considered on a case-by-case basis to rule out aneurysm.
3) An LP should be done to rule out subarachnoid hemorrhage when exertional pain is severe and occurs suddenly. *But the performance of an LP must await the performance and results of a CT scan, with and without enhancement, or MRI.*

4. Principles of treatment

a. The provoking effort must be curtailed until a diagnosis is established
b. Pharmacological measures are generally indicated

 c. Attacks that occur predictably and occasionally can be treated by therapies given just before exertion, or if they occur unpredictably and frequently, through preventive therapy.

5. Specifics of treatment

 a. *Symptomatic pharmacotherapy.* Symptomatic treatment can be administered 1–2 hours *before* the anticipated exertional event. Medications useful in this setting include:

  (1) Indomethacin 25–50 mg

  (2) Ergot derivatives (methysergide, methylergonovine, ergotamine tartrate)

  (3) Isometheptene (Midrin, etc.)

  (4) Propranolol (20–40 mg)

 b. Preventive pharmacotherapy:

  (1) Indomethacin

  (2) β-adrenegic blocking agents

  (3) Methysergide/methylergonovine

  (4) Other migraine preventive agents

 c. *Lumbar puncture.* An LP, for reasons not yet apparent, may be effective in terminating the attacks for a period of time.

B. Coital Headache/Headaches Associated with Sexual Activity/Benign Sexual Headaches

1. Introduction

Headache may occur just prior to, at the time of, or just after orgasm. It is rarely if ever of psychological origin. The syndrome appears to correlate poorly with degree of physical exertion or sexual excitement and generally occurs infrequently and unpredictably. It has been reported after masturbation. The headache usually ceases if sexual activity stops. Men appear more vulnerable to the syndrome than women (4:1).

2. Key clinical features

Three patterns of bilateral headache may occur.

 a. *Sudden onset.* In 70% of cases, the headache begins just before, during, or just after orgasm. The headache is of severe intensity, usually frontal or occipital, and may be throbbing. Explosive attacks are reported. The duration of pain is usually several hours, and a low-grade discomfort may persist. Accompaniments are rare, but confusion, palpitations, and vomiting have been reported. A prior or family history of migraine has been reported in about 25% of patients.

b. *Subacute, crescendo headache.* The second pattern is present in about 25% of cases and usually has onset much earlier than orgasm. It often increases in intensity until the time of orgasm. It has a dull, aching quality and is frequently located in the occiput.

c. *Postural headache.* The third and least common form of coital headache is a postural headache, occurring in the suboccipital area, markedly accentuated when the patient is upright. It is more frequently associated with nausea and vomiting than the other forms. Low CSF pressure has been confirmed in at least one instance. The syndrome may result from a tear in the dura caused by exertion and clinically resembles a post-LP headache.

3. Diagnosis

Same as II. A. 3.

4. Principles of treatment

Same as II. A. 4. and II. A. 5.

Also, if low CSF pressure is suspected, assessment and treatment are according to guidelines for low-pressure headache (see Chapter 15).

C. Hemicrania Continua
1. Introduction

In 1984, Sjaastad and Spierings described an unusual headache syndrome which was distinctly and completely responsive to indomethacin. Its main features included a continuous unilateral headache that was moderate to severe in intensity. Frequently, patients experienced a jabbing, icepick-like phenomenon, provoked by physical exertion.

Many patients evolve from episodic hemicranial pain with migrainous features to a continuous lateralized pain. Icepick components are present in almost half of cases (Raskin, 1988).

2. Key clinical features

a. The key clinical features are:
1. Unilateral headache/variable location
2. Continuous pattern
3. Moderate to severe intensity
4. Few attack-related autonomic features
5. Absence of reliable precipitating features

6. Complete responsiveness to indomethacin
7. Female to male ratio—5:1
8. Mean age of onset—35.2 (11–58 years)
9. Mean duration of illness—10.5 years
10. Head trauma present in 22% of cases

b. Other clinical features include:
1. Nocturnal awakening
2. Photophobia
3. Menstrual aggravation

3. Diagnosis

a. Same as II. A. 4.
b. The response to indomethacin is diagnostic

4. Principles of treatment

Same as II. A. 4., II. A. 5

D. Chronic Paroxysmal Hemicrania (CPH)

1. Introduction

Many consider CPH a variant of cluster headache. It was first described by Sjaastad and Dale in 1974. The condition occurs primarily in women and sometimes young girls, and the attacks, unlike cluster headaches, may be precipitated by flexion and occasionally by rotation of the neck.

2. Key clinical features

a. Pain is unilateral and localized to the temple, forehead, ear, eye, or occipital regions
b. Attacks of pain last 5–30 minutes, averaging 10–15 minutes (by comparison to cluster headache, which has a mean duration of 45 minutes)
c. Attack frequency may be up to 15–30 per day, but average 10–15 attacks per day
d. Nocturnal awakening is reported
e. Autonomic symptoms, similar to those in cluster headache:
   1) tearing
   2) forehead perspiration
   3) conjunctival injection
   4) bradycardia/tachycardia
   5) rhinorrhea
   6) ptosis
   7) edema of eyelid
   8) pupillary changes
f. Headache can be provoked by movement in 10% of cases

g. Patients will frequently resort to excessive aspirin or OTC ibuprofen to control pain, perhaps due to the similarity in effect of indomethacin.

3. Establishing the diagnosis

Cluster headache is the most important differential diagnostic possibility. Attacks of CPH, as in cluster headache, have been mimicked by intracranial disease of either a structural or infiltrative infectious type, including aneurysm of ophthalmic artery and pituitary tumor.

The following studies are recommended:

a. CT scan with and without contrast, and preferably an MRI
b. LP in questionable cases
c. MRI angiogram or arteriogram in resistant cases
d. Evaluation of the eyes for pathology, including glaucoma, orbital pseudotumor, etc.

Indomethacin is reliable and effective and can be used for diagnostic purposes. Pursuit of the neurological workup often can await a trial of treatment.

4. Specifics of treatment

a. Indomethacin, 25–50 mg t.i.d.
b. Corticosteroids, if necessary

15

CSF Hypotension
(Low-Pressure Headache)

I. Introduction
Headache secondary to low cerebrospinal fluid pressure is most commonly a consequence of lumbar puncture performed for diagnostic or therapeutic purposes. The syndrome may produce headache that goes undiagnosed for an extended period.

II. Key Clinical Features
A. Frontal headache occurring or accentuated within 15 minutes of assuming upright position and ameliorated within 15 minutes of recumbency
B. Nausea and vomiting
C. Dizziness
D. Mild stiff neck
E. Occasional bradycardia

III. Mechanism
The proposed mechanism of intracranial hypotension includes one or more of the following:
A. Lumbar puncture with persistent CSF leak
B. Leakage from dural tear
  1. Head/neck trauma
  2. Opening of cranial vault
  3. Spontaneous CSF leakage
  4. ? Exertion-induced tear (orgasmic headache? See Chapter 14)
C. Decreased CSF production
  1. Dehydration
  2. Diabetic ketoacidosis
  3. Uremia
  4. Severe infection
D. CSF hyperabsorption (idiopathic intracranial hypotension)
E. Arnold Chiari malformation (Type I); has been associated with a low-pressure headache syndrome (see Khurana, 1991)

III. Diagnosis
A. The diagnosis is suspected in the presence of characteristic symptoms

    B. Other headaches associated with postural or exertional aggravation must be ruled out, including:
      1. Intracranial tumors
      2. Occipitocervical deformities (Arnold Chiari malformation, type I, etc.)
      3. Ventricular obstructive syndromes
      4. Exertional migraine
      5. Cervical disc disease
      6. Cranial sinus disease
      7. Cerebral vein thrombosis
      8. Subdural hematoma (can also occur as consequence of low pressure)
      9. Others
    C. CT scan/MRI of head and neck rule out intracranial or intraspinal disease if diagnosis is not apparent.
    D. Diagnosis is confirmed by LP demonstrating CSF pressure lower than 0–30 mm CSF by manometric measurement. (Low CSF pressure, as measured by lumbar puncture manometric evaluation, could result from an intraspinal obstruction above the lumbar space entered or from obstruction intracranially.) Also, failure to properly enter the subarachnoid space can result in overlooking abnormal pressure.
    E. Isotope cisternography with radioactive tracer to demonstrate:
      1. Leakage
      2. Rapid transport (hyperabsorption) via early visualization of kidneys and bladder
    F. Pantopaque myelography to demonstrate the presence of a dural tear not otherwise apparent.

III. Treatment

The treatment is directed at supportive measures and at the cause, if identified.

A. General Symptomatic Treatment
    1. Fluid replacement
    2. Bedrest
    3. Support hose
    4. Abdominal binder

B. Specific Treatment
    1. Treatment for primary disorder, if present
    2. Caffeine sodium benzoate infusion (caffeine causes constriction of cerebral vasculature; may increase CSF pressure)

    a. 500 mg (0.5 grams) given via syringe containing 25 mg of normal saline, via "slow push,"

    b. 500 mg added to D–5 lactated Ringer's solution (500 ml–1,000 ml) and administered intravenously over several hours or longer

    c. Careful monitoring for palpitations and other effects of caffeine is required. If a liter or more of fluid is given, monitor for fluid overload, electrolyte imbalance, etc.

3. If the aforementioned treatments fail, epidural blood patching, reported successful with and without evidence of tear/leakage, becomes standard treatment for the syndrome

4. Surgical repair is necessary when a significant dural rent is identified

16

Idiopathic Intracranial Hypertension (Pseudotumor Cerebri, Benign Intracranial Hypertension)

I. Introduction

Pseudotumor cerebri, as this condition was formerly and best known, is characterized by increased intracranial pressure of uncertain and obscure etiology. It is associated with several symptoms, the most consistent of which is headache. The condition occurs in the absence of intracranial structural lesions and primarily affects overweight women. In the general population, the overall incidence of the condition is one per 100,000, whereas the incidence within a population of obese women of childbearing age is 19 per 100,000. Women more than men (ratio of 8:1) suffer from the illness. The average age of onset is 29–30 years.

II. Key Clinical Features
A. Primary Symptoms
The primary symptoms include:

1. Generalized, usually frontal headache, accompanied by papilledema. The headache is often associated with a postural component but is otherwise nonspecific in form. It may have migrainous or tension-type (migraine variant) features. It frequently persists even after pressure reduction occurs.
2. Nausea and vomiting
3. Progressive visual loss if sustained, unrelieved papilledema occurs
4. Occasional cranial nerve VI paresis
5. Dizziness and unsteadiness of gait, possibly related to postural hypotension
6. Stiff neck
7. Pulsatile tinnitus (may improve with ipsilateral, internal jugular vein compression and/or lumbar puncture)

B. Clinical Findings
Major clinical findings include:

1. Papilledema (present in over 90% of patients)
2. Visual findings may include:
   a. Enlargement of the physiological blind spot

b. Persistent blurring and moderate to severe reduction in visual acuity
c. Constriction of the visual fields
d. Inferonasal visual field defects

3. Confirmation of elevated pressure, over 200 (some authorities believe 250) mm of H_2O on manometric reading during a lumbar puncture

III. Mechanism

The mechanism of pseudotumor cerebri is unknown. Currently, it is believed due to increased flow resistance in the arachnoid villi and/or increase in dural sinus pressure. (The original case was the result of lateral venous thrombosis, thus initially called *otitic hydrocephalus*).

Other changes may include cerebral vasomotor instability, a loss of cerebrovascular regulation, and vasomotor instability (Raskin, 1988).

IV. Diagnosis
A. Making the Diagnosis
The diagnosis is established by:

1. Ruling out other causes of increased intracranial pressure and papilledema:
   a. Obstructive hydrocephalus
   b. Cerebral edema
   c. Cerebral vein thrombosis
   d. Vasculitis
   e. Intracranial mass: tumor, AVM
   f. Infectious/infiltrative CNS disease
2. Confirming elevation by the performance of lumbar puncture and manometric measurements

B. Other Diagnostic Considerations
1. Most diagnostic tests are normal; delayed VEP latency of P-100 is present in some cases.
2. CT scan is generally normal, but slightly enlarged or diminished ventricles have been noted; MRI and MRA may reveal venous occlusive disease, if present.
3. Evidence of other conditions possibly related may be present. These include:
   a. Endocrine abnormalities
      1) Hypocortisolism
      2) Hypoparathyroidism
      3) Other
   b. Hyper/hypovitaminosis

    c. Antibiotic treatment

    d. Hematological abnormalities

    e. Toxic exposure

    f. Danazol (danocrine) use

V. Principles of Treatment
A. Treatment is directed at:
  1. Reducing increased intracranial pressure

  2. Protecting vision

  3. Treating headache

B. Reduction of pressure via the following:
  1. Acetazolamide (Diamox)

  2. Diuretics

  3. Steroids (used less now than in the past)

  4. Repetitive lumbar punctures to maintain reduced pressure

C. For resistant cases of increased intracranial pressure:
  1. Optic nerve sheath decompression to improve and protect visual function

  2. Shunt procedures

D. Headache control:
  1. Drugs used to control migraine and its variants

  2. Analgesics

VI. Special Considerations
1. Obesity in females is the most apparent predisposing factor.

2. The most common visual disturbance is transient visual obscuration (loss of vision usually lasting for a few seconds). Permanent visual impairment occurs with chronic papilledema.

3. Disc swelling is poorly correlated to increased intracranial pressure.

4. Delayed visual evoked responses may be the most important neurodiagnostic test, other than lumbar puncture.

5. If gliosis develops in the optic nerve, ophthalmoscopic visualization for increased intracranial pressure is no longer reliable. Regular ophthalmological evaluations and visual field examinations are required to document visual function accurately.

6. Headache does not necessarily abate when pressure is reduced.

7. While papilledema is present in most patients, it is not present in all patients with pseudotumor cerebri. Reliance on a

lumbar puncture and manometric readings is necessary in suspected cases, *even in the absence of papilledema.*

8. Symptoms persist in 25% of cases, which become chronic and associated with asthenia, memory dysfunction, and/or persistent headache.

17

The Neck and Headache: Cervicogenic Headache

I. Introduction

Controversy surrounds the role of cervical spine pathology and the development of headache. The scope of this book does not allow a detailed involvement in this controversy. Instead, an overview of cause and treatment considerations will be offered.

In general, there are but a few headache disorders that do not bring with them accompanying neck pain. Conversely, most neck pain disorders with identifiable pathology are associated with elements of headache, some of which occur in the orbital, temporal, and frontal regions.

II. Anatomy, Physiology, and Possible Mechanisms

(For pain pathways of head and neck, see Chapter 3.)

A. Potential anatomical sources of headache within the cervical spine:
   1. Vertebral column
      a. Apophyseal joint
      b. Intervertebral disc
      c. Spinous ligaments
      d. Periosteum
   2. Cervical muscles
   3. Cervical nerves and roots, other soft tissues
   4. Vertebral arteries
B. Referred pain (to neck, vertex, frontal, orbital regions) might be the result of the following:
   1. Stimulation of the C1 sensory root
   2. Compression, inflammation, or irritation of the C2 sensory root or occipital nerves, zygapophyseal joints, etc.
   3. Stimulation of the upper cervical roots (overlap nucleus caudalis of the trigeminal system)
   4. Irritation of the tentorial nerves
   5. Spasm/tension in neck muscles
   6. Referred or muscle pain in the neck from migraine mechanisms in rostral regions

Fiber systems from C1, C2, and C3 may communicate with terminal branches of the supraorbital nerve and explain the fre-

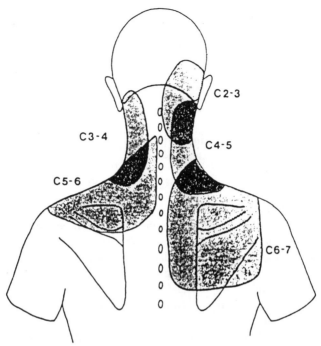

Figure 17.1. A composite map of the results in all volunteers depicting the putative characteristic distribution of pain from zygapophyseal joints at segments C2-3 to C6-7. (From Dwyer A, Aprill C, Bogduk N. Cervical zygapophyseal joint patterns I: A study in normal volunteers. *Spine* 15:453–457, 1990.)

quent association of orbital frontal pain in patients with neck injury or presumed pathology (Bogduk, 1981).

Figure 17.1 demonstrates a map of the distribution of pain from zygapophyseal joints at segments C2–C3 to C6–C7, as reported by Dwyer and associates (Dwyer, et al., 1990).

III. Clinical Conditions That Can Cause Headache and Neck Pain

A. Migraine
B. Occipital nerve neuralgia
C. Anomalies of the craniocervical junction
   1. Basilar invagination
   2. Arnold-Chiari malformation, type I
   3. Congenital atlantoaxial dislocation
   4. Dandy-Walker syndrome

     5. Occipitalization of the axis
     6. Other
  D. Craniocervical disease
     1. Tumor
     2. Neurofibroma
     3. Infection
     4. Paget's disease
     5. Others
  E. Arthritis/ankylosing spondylitis
  F. Cervical disc or root disease
  G. Trauma
  H. Others

IV. Key Clinical Features

A variety of pain patterns can arise from cervical disease, including:

A. Neuralgic or neuralgic-like syndromes
B. Nonspecific neck aching
C. "Muscular," myofascial pain
D. Generalized, nonspecific pain, often a prelude to a frank migraine attack

Occipital pain may arise as a component of transformational migraine or cluster headache. Neck pathology may, like pain arising from peripheral trigeminal distribution, activate true migraine (Winston, 1987).

V. The Diagnosis

A. The history and physical examination
B. Cervical spine x-rays
C. C-cord MRI/CT scan
D. EMG (not generally helpful in high neck regions)
E. Diagnostic nerve blocking (occipital nerve, zygapophyseal, facet joints, C2 and C3 nerves, etc.) (See Bovim, 1992a)

VI. Treatment

The treatment of neck pain with or without headache must take into account the general broad categories of illness described above as well as the overall approach to treating head pain. Specific pathological disorders of the neck must be addressed appropriately. The following therapeutic methods are available:

A. Pharmacotherapy, using drugs generally effective for migraine, neuralgic syndromes, etc.
B. Trigger point, zygapophyseal, facet joint, and occipital nerve blocking

C. Treating specific organic conditions, if identified
D. Conservative physical medicine measures, including:
   1. Physical therapy
   2. Transneural stimulation (TNS)
   3. Traction (can aggravate headache and neck pain)
   4. Biofeedback
E. Surgery (See Bovim, 1992b)

VII. Suggested Criteria for Suboccipital Blocking Procedures

A. The presence of persistent neck pain following appropriate conservative therapy
B. The onset of pain following neck or head injury
C. The identified or suspected presence of cervico-occipital pathology
D. Provocation of headache by neck movement
E. When localized pain foci are clearly present in the occipitocervical junction

VIII. Special Considerations

Much more must be understood before a definitive relationship between cervical pathology and persistent headache can be defined fully. Persistent, nociceptive, afferent input to the nucleus caudalis could play a primary role in the development of headache. Supraspinal, vascular, and other input to the system may be important as well. *Post-traumatic migraine* following neck injury in patients not previously experiencing headache supports the possibility that injuries to the neck region may result in provocation of migraine. Chronic afferent stimulation may also recruit sufficient activity within the pain modulating zone so as to "deplete" or "fatigue" this system, thereby also producing pain phenomena. In addition, referral of pain from head to neck or "release" of muscle tone mechanisms in the neck from brainstem control during physiological disturbances such as migraine might, speculatively, account for the overlap of symptoms.

In short, a headache is usually more than just a pain in the neck, but surely, it is that too!

Appendix A

LIST OF COMMON TRADE AND GENERIC NAMES

Trade	Generic
Adapin	Doxepin HCl
Advil	Ibuprofen 200 mg
Aldactone	Spironolactone
Anaprox	Naproxyn sodium (275 mg)
Anaprox DS	Naproxyn sodium (550 mg)
Anexsia 7.5	Hydrocodone bitartrate 7.5 mg/Acetaminophen 650 mg
Anexsia	Hydrocodone bitartrate 5 mg/Acetaminophen 500 mg
Antivert	Meclizine
Aristocort (tablets)	Triamcinolone
Asendin	Amoxapine
Atarax	Hydroxyzine HCl
Ativan	Lorazepam
Axotal	Butalbital 50 mg/Aspirin 650 mg
B & O Supprettes (suppositories)	No. 15 A: Opium 30 mg and Belladonna extract 16.2 mg
	No. 16 A: Opium 60 mg and Belladonna extract 16.2 mg
B-A-C	Butalbital 50 mg/Aspirin 650 mg/Caffeine 40 mg
Bancap HC	Hydrocodone bitartrate 5 mg/Acetaminophen 500 mg
Belladenal-S	Phenobarbital 50 mg/Bellafoline 0.25 mg/Tartrazine
Bellergal-S	Phenobarbital 40 mg/Bellafoline 0.2 mg Ergotamine tartrate 0.6 mg
Benadryl	Diphenhydramine
Bonine	Meclizine
Buprenex (injectable)	Buprenorphine HCl
BuSpar	Buspirone HCl
Butisol Sodium	Butabarbital sodium
Cafergot (suppositories)	Ergotamine tartrate 2 mg/Caffeine 100 mg
Cafergot (tablets)	Ergotamine tartrate 1 mg/Caffeine 100 mg
Calan	Verapamil
Calan SR	Verapamil
Captopril	Capoten
Cardene	Nicardipine HCl
Cardizem	Diltiazem
Cardizem SR	Diltiazem
Catapres	Clonidine
Celestone (tablets)	Betamethasone
Centrax	Prazepam
Clinoril	Sulindac
Co-Gesic	Hydrocodone bitartrate 5 mg/Acetaminophen 500 mg
Compazine	Prochloroperazine
Corgard	Nadolol
Cortone (tablets)	Cortisone acetate
D.H.E. 45	Dihydroergotamine mesylate

LIST OF COMMON TRADE AND GENERIC NAMES (CONTINUED)

Trade	Generic
Damason-P	Hydrocodone bitartrate 5 mg/Aspirin 224 mg/ Caffeine 32 mg
Darvocet-N 100	Propoxyphene napsylate 100 mg/ Acetaminophen 650 mg
Darvocet-N 50	Propoxyphene napsylate 50 mg/Acetaminophen 325 mg
Darvon Compound	Propoxyphene HCl 32 mg/Aspirin 389 mg/ Caffeine 32.4 mg
Darvon Compound-65	Propoxyphene HCl 65 mg/Aspirin 389 mg/ Caffeine 32.4 mg
Darvon with A.S.A	Propoxyphene HCl 65 mg/Aspirin 325 mg
Darvon-N	Propoxyphene napsylate
Darvon-N with A.S.A	Propoxyphene napsylate 100 mg/Aspirin 325 mg
Decadron (tablets and suspension)	Dexamethasone
Deltasone (tablets)	Prednisone
Demerol (tablets/injectable)	Meperidine HCl
Depakote	Divalproex sodium
Depo-Medrol (suspension)	Methylprednisolone acetate
Desyrel	Trazodone
Diamox	Acetazolamide
Dilantin	Phenytoin
Dilaudid	Hydromorphone HCl
Dolophine HCl (tablets)	Methadone HCl
Dramamine	Dimenhydrinate
DuoCet	Hydrocodone bitartrate 5 mg/Acetaminophen 500 mg
Elavil	Amitriptyline HCl
Empirin with Codeine #2	Codeine 15 mg/Aspirin 325 mg
Empirin with Codeine #3	Codeine 30 mg/Aspirin 325 mg
Empirin with Codeine #4	Codeine 60 mg/Aspirin 325 mg
Endep	Amitriptyline HCl
Ergomar (sl tablets)	Ergotamine tartrate 2 mg
Ergostat (sl tablets)	Ergotamine tartrate 2 mg
Esgic	Butalbital 50 mg/Acetaminophen 325 mg/ Caffeine 40 mg
Esgic with codeine	Butalbital 50 mg/Acetaminophen 325 mg/ Caffeine 40 mg/Codeine 30 mg
Eskalith	Lithium carbonate
Eskalith CR	Lithium carbonate
Etrafon	Amitriptyline HCl (10 mg, 25 mg)/ Perphenazine (2 mg, 4 mg)
Fiogesic	Pseudoephedrine HCl 30 mg/Aspirin 325 mg
Fioricet	Butalbital 50 mg/Acetaminophen 325 mg/ Caffeine 40 mg
Fiorinal	Butalbital 50 mg/Aspirin 325 mg/Caffeine 40 mg
Fiorinal with Codeine No. 3	Butalbital 50 mg/Aspirin 325 mg/Caffeine 40 mg/Codeine 30 mg
Flexeril	Cyclobenzaprine
Hydrocet	Hydrocodone bitartrate 5 mg/Acetaminophen 500 mg
Hydrocortone (tablets)	Hydrocortisone

LIST OF COMMON TRADE AND GENERIC NAMES (CONTINUED)

Trade	Generic
Inderal	Propranolol
Inderal LA	Propranolol
Indocin	Indomethacin
Isocom	Isometheptene mucate 65 mg/ Dichloralphenazone 100 mg/Acetaminophen 325 mg
Isoptin	Verapamil
Kenalog (suspension)	Triamcinolone acetonide
Klonopin	Clonazepam
Levo-Dromoran	Levorphanol tartrate
Librium	Chlordiazepoxide
Lidocaine 4% solution	Lidocaine HCl
Limbitrol	Chlordiazepoxide 5 mg/Amitriptyline HCl 12.5 mg
Limbitrol DS	Chlordiazepoxide 10 mg/Amitriptyline HCl 25 mg
Lioresal	Baclofen
Lithane	Lithium carbonate
Lithobid	Lithium carbonate
Lopressor	Metoprolol
Ludiomil	Maprotiline
Marcaine HCl	Bupivacaine HCl
Marplan	Isocarboxazid
Mebaral	Mephobarbital
Meclomen	Meclofenamate sodium
Medipren	Ibuprofen 200 mg
Medrol (tablets)	Methylprednisolone
Medrol Dosepak	Methylprednisolone
Mellaril	Thioridazine HCl
Mepergan (injectable)	Meperidine HCl/Promethazine HCl
Methergine	Methylergonovine maleate
Midol	Ibuprofen 200 mg
Midrin	Isometheptene mucate 65 mg/ Dichloralphenazone 100 mg/Acetaminophen 325 mg
Migralam	Isometheptene mucate 65 mg/Caffeine 100 mg/Acetaminophen 325 mg
Miltown	Meprobamate
MS Contin (tablets)	Morphine sulphate
MSIR (tablets/oral solution)	Morphine sulphate
Nalfon	Fenoprofen calcium
Naprosyn	Naproxyn
Narcan (injectable)	Naloxone HCl
Nardil	Phenelzine
Nembutal	Pentobarbital
Nembutal Sodium	Pentobarbital sodium
Norflex	Orphenadrine citrate
Norgesic	Orphenadrine citrate 25 mg/Aspirin 385 mg/ Caffeine 30 mg
Norgesic Forte	Orphenadrine citrate 50 mg/Aspirin 770 mg/ Caffeine 60 mg
Norpramin	Desipramine HCl
Nubain (injectable)	Nalbuphine HCl

LIST OF COMMON TRADE AND GENERIC NAMES (CONTINUED)

Trade	Generic
Numorphan (injectable, rectal suppositories)	Oxymorphan HCl
Nuprin	Ibuprofen 200 mg
Pamelor	Nortriptyline HCl
Pantopon (injectable)	Opium alkaloid hydrochlorides
Paraflex	Chlorzoxazone
Parafon Forte DSC	Chlorzoxazone
Parnate	Tranylcypromine
Paxipam	Halazepam
Pepto-Bismol	Bismuth subsalicylate
Percocet	Oxycodone 5 mg/Acetaminophen 325 mg
Percodan	Oxycodone HCl 4.5 mg/Oxycodone terephthalate 0.38 mg/Aspirin 325 mg
Percodan-Demi	Oxycodone HCl 2.25 mg/Oxycodone terephthalate 0.19 mg/Aspirin 325 mg
Percogesic	Phenyltoloxamine citrate 325 mg/ Acetaminophen 30 mg
Periactin	Cyproheptadine HCl
Persantine	Dipyridamole
Pertofrane	Desipramine HCl
Phenaphen #2	Acetaminophen 325 mg/Codeine 15 mg
Phenaphen #3	Acetaminophen 325 mg/Codeine 30 mg
Phenaphen #4	Acetaminophen 325 mg/Codeine 60 mg
Phenergan	Promethazine HCl
Phenobarbital	Phenobarbital
Phenobarbital sodium (injectable)	Phenobarbital
Phenobarbital Tablets	Phenobarbital
Phrenilin	Butalbital 50 mg/Acetaminophen 325 mg
Phrenilin Forte	Butalbital 50 mg/Acetaminophen 650 mg
Phrenilin with Codeine #3	Butalbital 50 mg/Acetaminophen 325 mg/ Codeine phosphate 30 mg
Ponstel	Mefenamic acid
Prolixin	Fluphenazine HCl
Prozac	Fluoxetine HCl
Reglan	Metoclopramide HCl
Robaxin	Methocarbamol
Robaxin-750	Methocarbamol
Roxanal 100 (oral solution)	Morphine sulphate
Roxanal SR (tablets/oral solution)	Morphine sulphate
Roxicet (tablets)	Oxycodone 5 mg/Acetaminophen 325 mg
Roxicodone (tablets and oral solution)	Oxycodone HCl
Salflex	Salsalate
Sansert	Methysergide maleate
Sectral	Acebutolol
Serax	Oxazepam
Sibelium	Flunarizine
Sinequan	Doxepin HCl
Skelaxin	Metaxalone
Soma	Carisoprodol

LIST OF COMMON TRADE AND GENERIC NAMES (CONTINUED)

Trade	Generic
Stadol (injectable/nasal spray)	Butorphanol tartrate
Surmontil	Trimipramine HCl
Synalgos-DC	Dihydrocodeine bitartrate 16 mg/Aspirin 356.4 mg/Caffeine 30 mg
Talacen	Pentazocine HCl 25 mg/Acetaminophen 650 mg
Talwin Compound	Pentazocine HCl 12.5 mg/Aspirin 325 mg
Talwin Nx	Pentazocine HCl 50 mg/Naloxone HCl 0.5 mg
Tegretol	Carbamazepine
Tenormin	Atenolol
Thorazine	Chlorpromazine
Tigan	Trimethobenzamide HCl
Tofranil	Imipramine HCl
Tofranil-PM	Imipramine HCl
Torecan	Thiethylperazine maleate
Transderm Scop	Scopolamine
Tranxene	Clorazepate
Trexan	Naltrexone
Triavil	Amitriptyline HCl (10 mg, 25 mg, 50 mg)/ Perphenazine (2 mg, 4 mg)
Trilafon	Perphenazine
Tylenol #2	Acetaminophen 300 mg/Codeine 15 mg
Tylenol #3	Acetaminophen 300 mg/Codeine 30 mg
Tylenol #4	Acetaminophen 300 mg/Codeine 60 mg
Tylox	Oxycodone 5 mg/Acetaminophen 500 mg
Valium	Diazepam
Valrelease	Diazepam
Vasotec	Enalapril maleate
Vicodin	Hydrocodone bitartrate 5 mg/Acetaminophen 500 mg
Vistaril	Hydroxyzine pamoate
Vivactil	Protriptyline HCl
Wellbutrin	Bupropion
Wigraine (suppositories)	Ergotamine tartrate 2 mg/Caffeine 100 mg/ Tartaric acid 21.5 mg
Wigraine (tablets)	Ergotamine tartrate 1 mg/Caffeine 100 mg
Wygesic	Propoxyphene HCl 65 mg/Acetaminophen 650 mg
Xanax	Alprazolam
Zydone	Hydrocodone bitartrate 5 mg/Acetaminophen 500 mg

Appendix B

SELECTED ESSENTIAL PHARMACOKINETICS OF COMMONLY USED HEADACHE DRUGS[a]

Drug	Route	Dosing Interval	Onset of Action	Duration of Action	Protein Binding (%)	Elimination Half-Life[b]	Route of Elimination
Acebutolol	PO	12–24 hr	1.5 hr	—	26	3–4 hr (8–13 hr)	30–40% renal/50–60% fecal
Acetaminophen	PO	4–6 hr	10–60 min	4–6 hr	<50	1.6–2.4 hr	Renal
Alprazolam	PO	8 hr	—	—	80	12–15 hr	Renal
Amitriptyline	PO	8–24 hr	2 wk	—	94.8	6–22 hr (18–44 hr)	Renal
Amobarbital	PO	6–12 hr	10–30 min	3–11 hr	—	20–25 hr	Renal
Amoxapine	PO	24 hr	<2 wk	—	90	8 hr (30 hr)	Renal
Aprobarbital	PO	8 hr	20–60 min	6–8 hr	20	14–40 hr	Renal
Atenolol	PO	24 hr	1 hr	24 hr	10	6–7 hr	70–80% renal/20–30% fecal
Baclofen	PO	8 hr	Hours to weeks	8 hr	30	2.5–4 hr	Renal
Buprenorphine	IM	6 hr	15 min	1–6 hr	96	1.2–7.2 hr	Renal
	IV	6 hr	<15 min	<6 hr			
Buspirone	PO	8 hr	—	—	95	2–3 hr	29–63% renal/18–38% fecal
Butabarbital	PO	6–8 hr	10–30 min	6–8 hr	—	34–42 hr	Renal
Butorphanol	IM	3–4 hr	<10 min	3–4 hr	80	3–4 hr	60–80% renal/11–14% fecal
Captopril	IV	3–4 hr	1 min	2–4 hr	25–35	1.9 hr	Renal
Carbamazepine	PO	8–12 hr	<15 min	2–6 hr	76	12–17 hr	72% renal/28% fecal
Carisoprodol	PO	6–12 hr	5–7 days	12–24 hr	—	8 hr	Renal
Chloral hydrate	PO	8 hr	<30 min	4–6 hr	—	8–11 hr	Renal/biliary
Chlordiazepoxide	PO	8–24 hr	1 hr	—	96–97	7–13 hr (5–10 hr; 48–76 hr)	Renal

SELECTED ESSENTIAL PHARMACOKINETICS OF COMMONLY USED HEADACHE DRUGS[a] (CONTINUED)

Drug	Route	Dosing Interval	Onset of Action	Duration of Action	Protein Binding (%)	Elimination Half-Life[b]	Route of Elimination
Chlormezanone	PO	6–8 hr	15–30 min	—	48	24 hr	Renal/biliary
Chlorpheniramine	PO	4–6 hr	30 min–1 hr	4–24 hr	69–72	12–43 hr	Renal
Chlorpromazine	IM	3–4 hr					
	PO	6–8 hr					
Chlorprothixene	IM	6–8 hr	30 min–1 hr	4–6 hr	95–98	23–37 hr	Renal/fecal
	PO	6–8 hr	10–30 min				
Chlorzoxazone	PO	6–8 hr	1 hr	3–4 hr	—	1 hr	Renal/fecal
Clomipramine	PO	24 hr	2–3 wk		98	19–37 hr (32 hr)	Renal
Clonazepam	PO	8 hr	1–2 hr	6–12 hr	86	18–50 hr	Renal/fecal
Clonidine	Patch	7 days	2–3 days	7 days	—		Renal
Clorazepate	PO	8–12 hr	30 min–1 hr	6–8 hr	—	7–20 hr	65% renal/20% biliary
	PO	6–24 hr			97.5	1–3 hr (5–10 hr; 48–76 hr)	Renal
Codeine	IM/SC	4–6 hr	15–30 min	4–6 hr		2.5–4 hr	Renal
	PO	4–6 hr	15–30 min	4–6 hr	<50		
Cyclobenzaprine	PO	8 hr	1 hr	12–24 hr	93	1–3 days	Renal
Cyproheptadine	PO	8 hr	30 min–1 hr	8–12 hr	—	—	65–75% renal/25–35% fecal
Desipramine	PO	8–24 hr	<2–3 wk		90	12–24 hr	Renal
Diazepam	IM	3–4 hr	15–30 min		97–99		Renal
	IV	3–4 hr	1–5 min	15–60 min			
	PO	6–12 hr	15–45 min			30–56 hr (5–10 hr; 48–76 hr)	
Dihydroergotamine	IM	1 hr	15–30 min	3–4 hr	90	21–32 hr	90% biliary/10% renal
	IV	1 hr	5–10 min				
Diltiazem	PO	6–8 hr	30 min		80	3.5 hr	Renal/biliary
Diphenhydramine	PO/IM/IV	4–6 hr	<1 h	4–6 hr	82	2.4–7 hr	Renal
Doxepin	PO	8–24 hr	2 wk		90	11–23 hr (34–68 hr)	Renal
Ergotamine	Inhal	5 min					Fecal
	PO, SL	0.5 hr	5 hr		—	21 hr	
Fluoxetine	PO		>4 wk	2–4 wk	95	2–3 days (7–9 days)	Renal
Fluphenazine hydrochloride	PO	12–24 hr	1 hr				Renal/fecal
	IM	6–8 hr		6–8 hr	80	17.5–15.8 hr	

Flurazepam	PO	6–8 hr	1 hr	1 hr	80	14.7–15.3 hr	Renal/fecal
Halazepam	PO	24 hr	15–45 min	7–8 hr	96.6	2–3 hr (47–100 hr)	Renal
		6–8 hr			97	14 hr (5–10 hr; 48–76 hr)	Renal
Hydrocodone	PO	4–6 hr	10–30 min	4–6 hr		3.8 hr	Renal
Hydromorphone	IM, SC	4–6 hr	15–30 min	4–5 hr			
	IV		<15 min	4–5 hr			
	PO	4–6 hr	30 min	4–5 hr		1.8–3.5 hr	Renal
Hydroxyzine	IM	4–6 hr	15–30 min	4–6 hr		3 hr	Biliary
Ibuprofen	PO	6 hr	30 min	4–6 hr	90–99	1.8–2 hr	Renal
Imipramine	IM	4–6 hr	2 wk		94.8	11–25 hr (12–24 hr)	Renal
	PO	6–24 hr	7–14 days		90	4.5 hr	
Indomethacin	IM	6–24 hr	10 min	4–6 hr	99	4.5 hr	60% renal/33% fecal
Ketorolac	PO	8–12 hr	20 min	6–8 hr			91% renal/6% fecal
	IM	6 hr	10–60 min	6–8 hr			
Levorphanol	IV	6–8 hr	60–90 min	6–8 hr		11 hr	Renal
	PO	6–8 hr	5–15 min	<3 hr	60–80	1.5–2 hr	Renal
Lidocaine	SC	6–8 hr	5–7 days	12–24 hr	0	14–30 hr	Renal
Lithium	IM		15–30 min	6–8 hr			
Lorazepam	IM	6–8 hr	15–20 min		85	12–18 hr	Renal
	IV				88	27–58 hr	60% renal/30% fecal
Maprotiline	PO	8–12 hr	6–10 days		99.8	3.3 hr	66% renal/33% fecal
Meclofenamate	PO	8–24 hr		2–4 hr	60	2.4–4 hr	Renal
Meperidine	IM, SC	6–8 hr	10–15 min	2–4 hr			
	IV	3–4 hr	1 min	2–4 hr			
	PO		15 min	10–16 hr		11–67 hr (81–117 hr)	Renal
Mephobarbital	PO	3–4 hr		10–16 hr		11–67 hr (81–117 hr)	Renal
		24 hr (seizure)	20–60 min				
Meprobamate	PO	6–8 hr (sed/hyp)	1–3 hr	4–6 hr	20	6–16 hr	Renal
Metaxalone	PO	6–8 hr	<1 hr	4–6 hr		2–3 hr	Renal
	PO	6–8 hr	<1 hr	4–6 hr		2–3 hr	Renal
Methadone	IM/SC	3–4 hr	10–20 min	4–6 hr	90	13–47 hr	Renal/fecal
	PO	3–4 hr	30–60 min	4–6 hr		0.9–2.2 hr	Renal/fecal
Methocarbamol	PO	6–8 hr	<30 min	6–8 hr			

SELECTED ESSENTIAL PHARMACOKINETICS OF COMMONLY USED HEADACHE DRUGS^a (CONTINUED)

Drug	Route	Dosing Interval	Onset of Action	Duration of Action	Protein Binding (%)	Elimination Half-Life^b	Route of Elimination
Methysergide	PO	6–24 hr	1–2 days	1–2 days		10 hr	Renal
Metoclopramide	IV	2–3 hr	1–3 min	1–2 hr	13–22	5–6 hr	80% renal/
	PO	6–8 hr					
Metoprolol	PO	8–12 hr	12 hr	—	10–12	3–7 hr	Renal
Morhine	Rectal	4 hr	<20–60 min	4–5 hr			
Morphine	IM	4 hr	<30–60 min				
	IV		<20 min	4–5 hr			
	PO	4 hr	<60 min	4–5 hr	33	1.5–2 hr	85–90% renal/7–10% fecal
Morphine (SR)	SC	4 hr	<50–90 min	4–5 hr			
	PO	8–12 hr	<60 min			8–12 hr	
Nadolol	PO	12–24 hr		24 hr	25	20–24 hr	Renal
Nalbuphine	IM, SC	3–6 hr	<15 min	3–6 hr	<60	5 hr	Biliary/renal
	IV	3–6 hr	2–3 min	3–6 hr			
Naproxen	PO	12 hr	2 hr	<7 hr	99	13 hr	Renal
Naproxen sodium	PO	6–8 hr	1 hr	<7 hr	>99	13 hr	Renal
Nortriptyline	PO	8–24 hr	2 wk	—	92	18–93 hr	Renal
Orphenadrine	IM/IV	12 hr					
	PO	12 hr	1 hr	4–6 hr		14 hr	Renal
Oxazepam	PO	6–8 hr			97.8	5–10 hr	Renal
Oxycodone	PO	6 hr	10–15 min	3–6 hr		2–3 hr	Renal
Oxymorphone	IM, SC	4–6 hr	10–15 min	3–6 hr		—	Renal
	IV	4–6 hr	5–10 min	3–6 hr			
	Rectal	4–6 hr	15–30 min	3–6 hr			
Pentazocine	IM, SC	3–4 hr	15–20 min	2 hr			
	IV	3–4 hr	2–3 min	1 hr			
	PO	4 hr	15–30 min	3–4 hr	60	2–3 hr	Renal
Pentobarbital	IM		10–25 min				
	IV	—	1 min	15 min			
	PO	6–8 hr	15–60 min	1–4 hr	35–45	35–50 hr	Renal
Perphenazine	IM	6 hr			High	—	
	PO	6–12 hr					Renal/fecal

Drug	Route						
Phenobarbital	IM	8–12 hr	—	—	20–45	81–117 hr	Renal
	IV	8–12 hr	5 min	4–6 hr	20–45	81–117 hr	Renal
	PO	8–12 hr (sed/hyp)	1 hr	10–12 hr			
Phenytoin	IV	8–12 hr	2–3 wk (sz)	—			Renal
	PO	6–24 hr	1–2 hr	—	89	7–29 hr	Renal
Prazepam	PO	8–24 hr	2–24 hr	—	97.5	1–2 hr (5–10 hr; 48–76 hr)	Renal/fecal
Prochlorperazine	IM	3–4 hr	10–20 min	3–4 hr			
	PO	6–8 hr	30–40 min	3–4 hr	80–90		Renal/fecal
	Rectal	12 hr	60 min	—			
Promethazine	IM	—	—	—			
	IV	—	3–5 min	—			
	PO	4–6 hr	20 min	4–12 hr			Renal/fecal
Propoxyphene	PO	4 hr	15–60 min	4–6 hr	—	6–12 hr	Renal
Propranolol	PO	6–12 hr	1–.5 hr	—	90	4 hr	Renal
Propranolol (LA)	PO	24 hr	—	—			Renal
Protriptyline	PO	6–8 hr	2 wk	—	92	67–89 hr	Renal
Salicylates	PO	4 hr	<30 min	3–6 hr	75–90	2–19 hr	Renal
Scopolamine	Patch	72 hr	4 hr	up to 72 hr			
Spironolactone	PO	24 hr	2 days	2–3 days	90	9–26 hr	Renal
Thiethylperazine	PO	8–24 hr	30 min	4 hr	High	20–40 hr	Renal/biliary
Thioridazine	PO	6–12 hr	1–6 hr	—	>80		Renal/fecal
Thiothixene	IM	6–12 hr	Days to weeks	—			
	PO	8–12 hr		—			Biliary
Thyroxine	PO	24 hr	3–5 days	7–10 days	—	6–7 days	Renal/biliary
Trazodone	PO	6 hr	1–4 wk	—	99	5–9 hr	70–75% renal/20–25% biliary
Triazolam	PO	24 hr		—	89–95	1.6–5.4 hr	Renal
Trifluoperazine	IM	4–6 hr	2–3 wk	—			Renal/fecal
	PO	12 hr			47–85		
Trimethobenzamide	PO	6–8 hr	10–40 min	3–4 hr	>80		Renal/biliary
Trimipramine	PO	6–24 hr	≥2 wk	1–2 days	—	9.1 hr	Renal/fecal
Valproic acid, divalproex	PO	8–12 hr	Few days to > 1 wk	—	>85	6–16 hr	Renal
Verapamil	PO	6–8 hr	1–2 hr	6–8 hr	90	2.8–12 hr	70% Renal/16% biliary
Verapamil (SR)	PO	12–24 hr	1–2 hr	12–24 hr			

[a] Modified from Compendium of Drug Therapy 1991–1992.
[b] Active metabolites.

General Suggested Reading

Basic Mechanisms of Headache, J Olesen, L Edvinson (Eds). Amsterdam, Elsevier Science Publishers, 1988.

Handbook of Clinical Neurology, FC Rose (Ed). Amsterdam, Elsevier Science Publishers, 1986, Volume 48.

Intractable headache: Inpatient and outpatient treatment strategies. SD Silberstein (Ed). *Neurology* (supp 2), March 1992.

Lance JW. *Mechanism and Management of Headache*, 4th Edition. London, Butterworth Scientific, 1982.

Markus DA. Migraine and tension-type headaches: The questionable validity of current classification systems. *Clin J Pain*, 8:28–36, 1992.

Neurologic Clinics: Headache. NT Mathew (Ed). November, 1990.

Olesen J. Classification and diagnostic criteria for headache disorders, cranial neuralgias, and headache pain. *Cephalalgia*, 8 (supp); 7:1–96, 1988.

Raskin NH. *Headache*, 2nd Edition. New York, Churchill Livingstone, 1988.

Saper JR. Changing perspectives on chronic headache. *Clin J Pain*, 2:19–28, 1986.

Saper JR. *Headache Disorders: Current Concepts and Treatment Strategies*, Littleton, Massachusetts, Wright-PSG Publishers, 1983.

Suggested Readings

Chapter 1

Linet MS, Stewart WF, Celentano DE, et al. An epidemiological study of headache among adolescents and young adults. *JAMA*, 261:2211–2216, 1989.

Olesen J. The classification and diagnosis of headache disorders. (In) *Neurologic Clinics*: NT Mathew (Ed). Pgs 793–799, November, 1990.

Ziegler DK. Headache: Public health problem. (In) *Neurologic Clinics*: NT Mathew (Ed). Pg 781–792, November, 1990.

Chapter 2

See standard texts (Suggested Reading List)

vanDusseldorp M, Katan MB. Headache caused by caffeine withdrawal among moderate coffee drinkers switched from ordinary to decaffeinated coffee: A 12-week, double-blind study. *Brit Med J*, 300:1558–1559, 1990.

Chapter 3

Bogduk N. The clinical anatomy of the cervical dorsal rami. *Spine*, 7:319–330, 1982.

Buzzi MG, Moskowitz MA. The antimigraine drug sumatriptan (GR43175) selectively blocks neurogenic plasma extravasation from blood vessels in dura mater. *Brit J Pharmacol*, 99:202–206, 1990.

Goadsby PJ, Zagami AS, Lambert GA. Neuroprocessing of craniovascular pain: A synthesis of the central structures involved in migraine. *Headache*, 31:365–371, 1991.

Moskowitz MA. Basic mechanisms in vascular headache. (In) *Neurologic Clinics*: NT Mathew (Ed). Pgs 801–815, November, 1990.

Olesen J. Clinical and pathophysiological observations in migraine and tension-type headache explained by integration of vascular, supraspinal, and myofascial inputs. *Pain*, 46:125–133, 1991.

Raskin NH. Serotonin receptors and headache. *New Engl J Med*, 325:353–354, 1991.

Raskin NH, Hosobuchi Y, Lamb S. Headache may arise from perturbation of brain. *Headache*, 27:416–420, 1987.

Saito K, Markowitz S, Moskowitz MA. Ergot alkaloids block neurogenic extravasation in dura mater: Proposed action in vascular headaches. *Ann Neurol*, 24:732–737, 1988.

Sessle BJ, Hu JW, Amano N, Zhong G. The convergence of cutaneous, tooth pulp, visceral, neck, and muscle afferents onto nociceptive and non-nociceptive neurons in trigeminal subnucleus caudalis (medullary dorsal horn) and its implications for referred pain. *Pain*, 27:219–235, 1986.

Silberstein SD. Advances in understanding the pathophysiology of headache. *Neurology*, 42 (supp 2):6–10, 1992.

Welch KMA, Andrea GD, Tepley N, et al. The concept of migraine as a state of central neuronal hyperexcitability. (In) *Neurologic Clinics*: Headache. NT Mathew (Ed). Pgs 817–828, 1990.

Chapter 4

Bindoff LA, Hezeltine D. Unilateral facial pain in patients with lung cancer: Referred pain via the vagus? *Lancet*, 1:812–825, 1988.

Cant RS, Daniel FI. Glossopharyngeal neuralgia in a child. *Arch Neurol*, 43:301–302, 1986.

Caplan L. Intracerebral hemorrhage revisited. *Neurology*, 38:624–627, 1988.

Cole AJ, Aube M. Migraine with vasospasm and delayed intracerebral hemorrhage. *Arch Neurol*, 47:53–56, 1990.

Cox LK, Bertorini T, Lassiter RE. Headaches due to spontaneous internal carotid artery dissection: Magnetic resonance imaging evaluation followup. *Headache*, 31:12–16, 1991.

Day JW, Raskin NH. Thunderclap headache: Symptom of unruptured cerebral aneurysm. *Lancet*, 2:1247–1248, 1986.

DeAngelis LM, Payne R. Lymphomatous meningitis presenting as atypical cluster headache. *Pain*, 30:211–216, 1987.

Druce HM, Slavin RG. Sinusitis: Critical need for further study. *J Allergy Clin Immunol*, 88:675–677, 1991.

Dwyer A, Aprill C, Bogduk N. Cervical zygapophyseal joint pain patterns I: A study in normal volunteers. *Spine*, 15:453–457, 1990.

Fisher CM. The headache and pain of spontaneous carotid dissection. *Headache*, 22:660–665, 1982.

Goldstein J. Headache and acquired immunodeficiency disorder. (In) *Neurologic Clinics*: NT Mathew (Ed). Pgs 947–960, November, 1990.

Halperin JJ, Volkman DJ, Wu P. Central nervous system abnormalities and lyme neuroborrelios. *Neurology*, 41:1571–1582, 1991.

Hannerz J. A case of parasellar meningioma mimicking cluster headache. *Cephalalgia*, 9:265–269, 1989.

Hannerz J. Recurrent Tolosa-Hunt syndrome. *Cephalalgia*, 12:45–51, 1992.

Harling DW, Peatfield RC, Van Hille PTE, et al. Thunderclap headache: Is it migraine? *Cephalalgia*, 9:87–90, 1989.

Khurana RK. Headache spectrum and Arnold-Chiari malformation. *Headache*, 31:151–155, 1991.

Marcelis J, Silberstein SD. Spontaneous low cerebral spinal fluid pressure headache. *Headache*, 30:192–196, 1990.

Metzer WS. Trigeminal neuralgia secondary to tumor with normal exam, responsive to carbamazepine. *Headache*, 31:164–166, 1991.

Nightingale S, Williams B. Hind brain hernia headache. *Lancet*, 1:731–734, 1987.

Raskin NH, Howard MW, Aaronfield WK. Headache as the leading symptom of thoracic outlet syndrome. *Headache*, 25:208–210, 1985.

Reik L, Steere AC, Bartenagen NH, et al. Neurologic abnormalities of lyme disease. *Medicine*, 58:281–294, 1979.

Rond R, Keane JR. The minor symptoms of increased intracranial pressure: 101 patients with benign intracranial hypertension. *Neurology*, 38:1461–1464, 1988.

Rothrock JF, Lim V, Press G, Gosink B. Serial magnetic resonance and carotid duplex examinations in the management of carotid dissection. *Neurology*, 38:686–692, 1989.

Shankland WE II. Ernest syndrome (insertion tendonosis of the stylomandibular ligament) as a cause for craniomandibular pain: Diagnosis, treatment, and report of two patients. *J Neurol & Orthopedic Med & Surg*, 8:253–257, 1987.

Sicuteri F, Nicolodi M, Fusco BM, et al. Idiopathic headache as a possible risk factor for phantom tooth pain. *Headache*, 31:577–581, 1991.

Silvestrini M, Cupini LM, Calabresi P, et al. Migraine with aura-like syndrome due to arteriovenous malformation. The clinical value of transcranial Doppler in early diagnosis. *Cephalalgia*, 12:115–119, 1992.

Smith RG, Cherry JE. Traumatic Eagle's syndrome: Report of a case and review of the literature. *J Oral Maxillofacial Surg*, 46:606–609, 1988.

Wijdicks EFM, Kerkhoff H, Vangijn J. Long-term follow-up with 71 patients with thunderclap headache mimicking subarachnoid hemorrhage. *Lancet*, 2:68–69, 1988.

Winston AR. Whiplash and its relationship to migraine. *Headache*, 27:452–457, 1987.

Chapter 5

Ayd FJ Jr. Guides for safe and effective use of combined tricyclic MAOI therapy. *International Drug Therapeutic Newsletter*, pg 14, 1979.

Ballenger JC, Post RM. Carbamazepine in alcohol withdrawal syndromes and schizophrenic psychoses. *Pharmacolog Bull*, 20:572–574, 1984.

Bernstein JE, Korman NJ, Bickers DR, et al. Topical capsaicin treatment of post-herpetic neuralgia. *J Am Acad Dermatol*, 21:265–270, 1989.

Boehnert MT, Lovejoy FH. The value of the QR restoration vs. the serum drug level in predicting seizures and ventricular arrhythmias after an acute overdose of tricyclic antidepressants. *New Engl J Med*, 313:474–479, 1985.

Buckoms AJ, Litman RE. Clonazepam in the treatment of neuralgic pain syndromes. *Psychosomatics*, 26:933–936, 1985.

Buzzi MG, Moskowitz MA. The antimigraine drug sumatriptan (GR43175) selectively blocks neurogenic plasma extravasation from blood vessels in dura mater. *Brit J Pharmacol*, 99:202–206, 1990.

Callaham MM, Raskin NH. A controlled study of dihydroergotamine in the treatment of acute migraine headache. *Headache*, 26:168–171, 1986.

Clary C, Schweitzer E. The treatment of MAOI hypertensive crisis with sublingual nifedipine. *Clin Psychiatry*, 48:249–250, 1987.

Diamond S, Dalessio DG. *The Practicing Physician's Approach to Headache*. 5th Edition. Baltimore, Williams & Wilkins, 1991.

Folks DG. Monoamine oxidase inhibitors: Re-appraisal of dietary considerations. *J Clin Pharmacol*, 3:246–252, 1983.

Fromm GH, Terrence CF, Chattha AS. Baclofen in the treatment of trigeminal neuralgia: Double-blind study and long-term follow-up. *Ann Neurol*, 15:240–244, 1984.

Goadsby PJ, Gundlach AL. Localization of ^{3}H-dihydroergotamine binding sites in the cat's central nervous system: Relevance to migraine. *Ann Neurol*, 29:91–94, 1991.

Goldstein J. Ergot pharmacology in alternative delivery systems for ergotamine derivatives. *Neurology*, 42 (supp 2):45–46, 1992.

Harrison WM, McGrath PJ, Stewart JW, Quitkin F. MAOIs and hypertensive crisis: The role of OTC drugs. *J Clin Psychiatry*, 50:64–65, 1989.

Herring R, Kuritzky A. Sodium valproate in the prophylactic treatment of migraine: A double-blind study vs. placebo. *Cephalalgia*, 12:81–84, 1992.

Jabbari B, Bryan GE, Marsh EE, et al. Incidence of seizures with tricyclic and tetracyclic antidepressants. *Arch Neurol*, 42:480–481, 1985.

King SA, Strange AJ. Benzodiazepine use by chronic pain patients. *Clin J Pain*, 6:147, 1990.

Lechin F, Vanderdigs B, Lechin ME, et al. Pimozide therapy for trigeminal neuralgia. *Arch Neurol*, 9:960–964, 1989.

Levenson ML, Lipsy RJ, Fuller DK. Adverse effects and drug interactions associated with fluoxetine therapy. *Ann Pharmacother*, 25:657–661, 1991.

Luckins A. A review of combined tricyclic and MAOI therapy. *Compr Psychiatry*, 18:221–230, 1977.

MacPhee GJA. Verapamil potentiates carbamazepine toxicity: A clinically important inhibitory interaction. *Lancet*, 1:700–703, 1986.

Mathew NT, Ali S. Valproate in the treatment of persistent chronic daily headache. An open-label study. *Headache*, 31:71–74, 1991.

Matthew RJ, Wilson WH. Caffeine-induced changes in cerebral circulation. *Stroke*, 16:814–817, 1985.

McQuay HJ, Carroll D, Watts PG, et al. Codeine 20 mg. increases pain relief from ibuprofen 400 mg. after third molar surgery. A repeat dosing comparison of ibuprofen in an ibuprofen-codeine combination. *Pain*, 37:7–13, 1989.

Peroutka SJ. The pharmacology of current antimigraine drugs. *Headache*, 30 (supp 1):5, 1990.

Portenoy RK. Chronic opioid therapy in non-malignant pain. *J Pain & Symptom Manage*, 5 (supp):46–61, 1990.

Raskin NH. Repetitive intravenous dihydroergotamine as therapy for intractable migraine. *Neurology*, 36:995–997, 1986.

Ries RK, Roy-Byrne PP, Ward NG, et al. Carbamazepine treatment for benzodiazepine withdrawal. *Am J Psychiatry*, 146:536–537, 1989.

Rumor MM, Schlichting DA. Clinical efficacy of antihistaminics as analgesics. *Pain*, 25:7–22, 1986.

Sandler D, Smith JC, Weinberg CR, et al. Analgesic use in chronic renal disease. *New Engl J Med* 320:1238–1243, 1989.

Saper JR. Daily chronic headache—Tension headaches, migraine, and combined headaches: The transformation concept. (In) *Drug-Induced Headache*, HC Diener and M Wilkinson (Eds). Berlin, Springer-Verlag, pgs 5–7, 1988.

Saper JR. Drug treatment of headache: Changing concepts and treatment strategies. *Semin Neurol*, 7:178–191, 1987.

Saper JR. Ergotamine dependency: A review. *Headache*, 27:435–458, 1987.

Saper JR. Chronic headache syndromes. *Neurol Clin*, 7:387–412, 1989.

Sechzer PG, Abel L. Post-spinal anesthesia headache treated with caffeine: Evaluation with demand method. Part I. *Curr Ther Res*, 24:307–312, 1978.

Silberstein SD, Shulman EA, Hopkins MM. Repetitive intravenous DHE in the treatment of refractory headache. *Headache*, 30:334–339, 1990.

Simone DA, Ochoa J. Early and late effects of prolonged topical capsaicin on cutaneous sensibility of neurogenic vasodilation in humans. *Pain*, 47:285–294, 1991.

Sorensen KV. Valproate: A new drug in migraine prophylaxis. *Acta Neurol Scandi*, 78:346–348, 1988.

Subcutaneous sumatriptan international study group. Treatment of migraine attacks with sumatriptan. *New Engl J Med* 1991;5:316–21.

The Capsaicin Study Group. Treatment of painful diabetic neuropathy with topical capsaicin. *Arch Int Med*, 151:2225–2229, 1991.

The Medical Letter. Ketorolac tromethamine, 32:79–81, 1990

The multinational oral sumatriptan and Cafergot comparative study group. A randomized, double-blind comparison of Cafergot and sumatriptan in the treatment of migraine. *European Neurology*, 1991;31:314–322.

The oral sumatriptan dose-defining study group. Sumatriptan—an oral dose-defining study. *European Neurology*, 1991;31:300–305.

The oral sumatriptan multiple-dose study group. Evaluation of a multiple-dose regimen of oral sumatriptan for the acute treatment of migraine. *European Neurology*, 1991;31:306–313. Tandan R, Lewis GA, Krvinski PB. Topical capsaicin in painful diabetic polyneuropathy: Controlled study with long-term follow-up. *Diabetic Care*, 15:8–14, 1992.

Ward N, Whitney C, Avery D, et al. The analgesic effects of caffeine in headache. *Pain*, 44:151–155, 1991.

Watson CPN, Evans RJ, Watt VR. Post-herpetic neuralgia and topical capsaicin. *Pain*, 33:333–340, 1988.

Westbrook L, Cicalar S, Wright H. The effectiveness of alprazolam in the treatment of chronic pain: Results of a preliminary study. *Clin J Pain*, 6:32–36, 1990.

White K, Simpson G. Combined use of MAOIs and tricyclics. *J Clin Psychiatry*, 45:67–69, 1984.

Chapter 6

Baumgartner CP, Wesseley P, Bingol C, et al. Long-term prognosis of analgesic withdrawal in patients with drug-induced headache. *Headache*, 29:510–514, 1989.

Belegrade MJ, Ling LJ, Schleevogt MB, et al. Comparison of single dose meperidine, butorphanol, and dihydroergotamine in treatment of vascular headache. *Neurology*, 39:590–592, 1989.

Bell R, Montoya D, Shuaib A, et al. A comparative trial of three agents in the treatment of acute migraine headache. *Amer Emerg Med*, 19:1079–1082, 1990.

Callaham M, Raskin NH. A controlled study of dihydroergotamine in the treatment of acute migraine headache. *Headache*, 26:168–171, 1986.

Diener HC, Dichgans J, Scholz E, et al. Analgesic-induced chronic headache. Long-term results of withdrawal therapy. *J Neurol*, 236:9–14, 1989.

Edmeads J. Emergency management of headache. *Headache*, 28:675–679, 1988.

Jones J, Sklar D, Dogherty J, et al. Randomized double-blind trial of intravenous prochlorperazine for the treatment of acute headache. *JAMA*, 261:1174–1176, 1989.

Lake AE, Saper JR, et al. Inpatient treatment for chronic daily headache: A prospective long-term outcome study. *Headache*, 30:299, 1990.

Neuman M, Demarez JP, Harmer JR, et al. Prevention of migraine attacks through use of dihydroergotamine. *Int J Clin Pharmacol Res*, 6:11–13, 1986.

Rapoport A, Weeks R, Sheftell F, et al. Analgesic rebound headache: Theoretical and practical implications. *Cephalalgia*, 5 (supp 3):448–450, 1985.

Rapoport AM, Silberstein SD. Emergency treatment of headache. *Neurology*. SD Silberstein (Ed), Supp 2, March, 1992.

Raskin NH. Repetitive intravenous dihydroergotamine as therapy for intractable migraine. *Neurology*, 36:995–997, 1986.

Saper JR, Jones JM. Ergotamine tartrate dependency: Features and possible mechanisms. *Clin Neuropharmacol*, 9:244–256, 1986.

Silberstein SD, Schulman EA, Hopkins MM. Repetitive intravenous DHE in the treatment of refractory headache. *Headache*, 30:334–339, 1990.

Silberstein SD, Silberstein JR. Analgesic/ergotamine rebound headache: Prognosis following detoxification and treatment with repetitive IV DHE. *Headache*, 32:352, 1992.

Chapter 7

Abramowicz M (ed). Transdermal estrogen. *Med Lett Drugs Ther*, 28:119–120, 1986.

Andermann F. Clinical features of migraine-epilepsy syndrome. (In) *Migraine and epilepsy*. Andermann F, Lugeresi E (Eds). Boston, Butterworth. Pgs 3–30, 1987.

Basser LS. The relation of migraine and epilepsy. *Brain*, 92:285–300, 1969.

Bickerstaff ER. Basilar artery migraine. (In) *Handbook of Clinical Neurology*, Vol. 48. FC Rose (Ed). Amsterdam, Elsevier Science Publishing, pgs 135–140, 1986.

Bickerstaff ER. Ophthalmoplegic migraine. *Rev Neurol*, 110:582–588, 1964.

Bickerstaff ER. The basilar artery and the migraine-epilepsy syndrome. *Royal Society Medical Proceedings*, 55:167–169, 1962.

Bradshaw P, Parsons M. Hemiplegic migraine: A clinical study. *Q J Med*, 34:65–85, 1965.

Bruyn GW. Complicated migraine. (In) *Handbook of Clinical Neurology*, Vol. 5. PJ Vincan, GW Bruyn (Eds). New York, John Wiley and Sons, pgs 59–95, 1968.

Bruyn GW. Migraine equivalents. (In) *Handbook of Clinical Neurology*, Vol. 48. FC Rose (Ed). Amsterdam, Elsevier Science Publishers, pgs 155–171, 1986.

Callahan N. The migraine syndrome in pregnancy. *Neurology*, 18:197–199, 1968.

Caplan L, Chedru F, Lheramitte F, Mayman C. Transient global amnesia and migraine. *Neurology*, 31:1167–1170, 1981.

Caplan L. Intracerebral hemorrhage revisited. *Neurology*, 38:624–627, 1988.

Cole AJ, Aube M. Migraine with vasospasm and delayed intracerebral hemorrhage. *Arch Neurol*, 47:53–56, 1990.

Dexter JD, Weitzman ED. The relationship of nocturnal headaches to sleep stage patterns. *Neurology*, 20:513–517, 1970.

Diener HC, Dichgans J, Scholz E, et al. Analgesic-induced chronic headache. Long-term results of withdrawal therapy. *J Neurol*, 236:9–14, 1989.

Ehyai A, Fenichel GM. The natural history of acute confusional migraine. *Arch Neurol*, 35:368–369, 1978.

Emery ES. Acute confusional state in migraine with children. *Pediatrics*, 60:110–114, 1977.

Fenichel GM. Migraine as a cause of benign paroxysmal vertigo of childhood. *J Pediatrs*, 71:114–115, 1967.

Fisher CM, Adams RD. Transient global amnesia. *Acta Neurol Scandinavia*, 40 (supp 9):1–83, 1964.

Fisher CM. Late life migraine accompaniments as a cause of unexplained transient ischemic attacks. *Can J Neurol Sci*, 7:9–17, 1980.

Fisher CM. Late life migraine accompaniments—further experience. *Stroke*, 17:1033–1042, 1986.

Fisher CM. Transient global amnesia: Precipitating activities and other observations. *Arch Neurol*, 39:605–608, 1982.

Gallucci M, Feliciani M, Martucci N, et al. Complicated migraine: An NMR and CT comparison. *Cephalalgia*, 5 (supp 3):376–377, 1985.

Gascon G, Barlow C. Juvenile migraine presenting as an acute confusional state. *Pediatrics*, 45:628–635, 1970.

Golden GS, French JS. Basilar artery migraine in young children. *Pediatrics*, 56:722–726, 1975.

Goldensohn ES. Paroxysmal and other features of the electroencephalogram in migraine. *Res Clin Stud Headache*, 4:118–128, 1976.

Harrison MJG. Hemiplegic migraine. *J Neurol Neurosurg Psychiatry*, 44:652–653, 1981.

Holroyd KA, Andrasik F. A cognitive-behavioral approach to recurrent tension and migraine headache. (In) PC Kendell (Ed) *Advances in Cognitive-Behavioral Research and Therapy*, New York, Academic, pgs 275–320, 1982.

Iniguez C, Pascual C, Pardo A, Martinez-Castrillo JC, et al. Antiphospholipid antibodies in migraine. *Headache*, 31:666–668, 1991.

Jacome DE. EEG features in basilar artery migraine. *Headache*, 27:80–83, 1987.

Jensen TS, Olivarius B, Kraft M, et al. Familial hemiplegic migraine—A reappraisal on a long-term follow-up study. *Cephalalgia*, 1:33–39, 1981.

Kuritzky A, Ziegler DK, Hassanein R. Vertigo motion sickness and migraine. *Headache*, 21:227–231, 1981.

Lance JW, Anthony M. Some clinical aspects of migraine. A prospective survey of 500 patients. *Arch Neurol*, 15:356–361, 1966.

Lanzi G, Balottin U, Ottolini A, et al. Cyclic vomiting and recurrent abdominal pains as migraine or epileptic equivalents. *Cephalalgia*, 3:115–118, 1983.

Lauritzen M, Trojaborg W, Olesen J. The eeg in common and classic migraine attacks. (In) *Advances in Migraine Research and Therapy*, FC Rose (Ed). New York, Raven Press, pgs 79–84, 1982.

Lee CH, Lance JW. Migraine stupor. *Headache*, 17:32–38, 1977.

Levine SR, Brey RL. Antiphospholipid antibodies and ischemic cerebrovascular disease. *Semina Neurol*, 11:329–338, 1991.

Olesen J. Some clinical features of the acute migraine attack. An analysis of 750 patients. *Headache*, 18:268–271, 1978.

Parrish RM, Stevens H. Familial hemiplegic migraine. *Minn Med*, 60:709–715, 1977.

Peatfield RC, Fozard JR, Rose FC. Drug treatment of migraine. (In) *Handbook of Clinical Neurology*, Vol. 48. FC Rose (Ed). Amsterdam, Elsevier Science Publishers, pgs 173–216, 1986.

Pfaffenrath V, Kommissari I, Pollmann W, et al. Cerebrovascular risk factors in migraine with prolonged aura and without aura. *Cephalalgia*, 11:257–161, 1991.

Rapoport A, Weeks R, Sheftell F, et al. Analgesic rebound headache: Theoretical and practical implications. *Cephalalgia*, 5 (supp 3):448–450, 1985.

Raskin NH, Schwartz RK. Icepick-like pain. *Neurology*, 30:203–205, 1980.

Shulman EA, Silberstein SD. Symptomatic and prophylactic treatment of migraine and tension-type headache. *Neurology*, 42 (supp 2):16–21, 1992.

Silberstein SD, Merriam GR. Estrogens, progestins, and headache. *Neurology*, 41:786–793, 1991.

Silberstein SD. The role of sex hormones in headache. *Neurology*, 42 (supp 2):37–42, 1992.

Silberstein SD. Twenty questions about headaches in children and adolescents. *Headache*, 30:716–724, 1990.

Solomon GD, Spaccavento LJ. Lateral medullary syndrome after basilar migraine. *Headache*, 22:171–172, 1982.

Somerville BW. Estrogen withdrawal migraine I and II. *Neurology*, 25:239–244, 245–250, 1975.

Somerville BW. The role of estradiol withdrawal in the etiology of menstrual migraine. *Neurology*, 22:355–365, 1972.

Sulkava R, Kovanen J. Locked-in syndrome with rapid recovery: A manifestation of basilar artery migraine? *Headache*, 23:238–239, 1983.

Teitjent GE. Migraine and antiphospholipid antibodies. *Cephalalgia*, 12:69–74, 1992.

Tinuper P, Cortelli P, Sacquengna T, Lugaresi E. Classic migraine attack complicated by confusional state: EEG and CT study. *Cephalalgia*, 5:63–68, 1985.

Tomsak RL, Jergens PB. Benign recurrent transient monocular blindness: A possible variant of acephalgic migraine. *Headache*, 27:66–69, 1987.

Watson P, Steele JC. Paroxysmal disequilibrium in the migraine syndrome of childhood. *Arch Otolaryngol*, 99:177–179, 1974.

Welch KMA, Darnley D, Simpkins RJ. The role of estrogen in migraine: A review and hypothesis. *Cephalalgia*, 4:227–236, 1984.

Whitty CWM. Familial hemiplegic migraine. (In) *Handbook of Clinical Neurology*, Vol. 48. FC Rose (Ed). Amsterdam, Elsevier Science Publishers, pgs 141–153, 1986.

Chapter 9

Andrasik F. Psychological and behavioral aspects of chronic headache. (In) *Neurologic Clinics*, NT Mathew (Ed). Pgs 961–976, November, 1990.

Baumgartner CP, Wesseley P, Bingol C, et al. Long-term prognosis of analgesic withdrawal in patients with drug-induced headache. *Headache*, 29:510–514, 1989.

Holroyd KA, Andrasik F. A cognitive-behavioral approach to recurrent tension and migraine headache. (In) *Advances in Cognitive-Behavioral Research and Therapy*, PC Kendell (Ed). New York, Academic, pgs 275–320, 1982.

Kudrow L. Paradoxical effects of frequent analgesic use. *Adv Neurol*, 33:335–341, 1982.

Lake AE III. Relaxation therapy and biofeedback in headache management. (In) *Help for Headaches*, JR Saper. Warner Books, New York, pgs 163–182, 1987.

Mathew NT, Reuveni U, Perez F. Transformed or evolutive migraine. *Headache*, 27:102–106, 1987.

Mathew NT. Drug-Induced Headache. (In) *Neurologic Clinics*, NT Mathew (Ed). Pgs 903–912, November, 1990.

Mathew NT, Stubits E, Nigam M. Transformation of migraine into daily chronic headache: Analysis of factors. *Headache*, 22:66–68, 1982.

Rapoport AM, Weeks RE, Sheftell FD, et al. The "analgesic washout period:" A critical variable in the evaluation of headache treatment efficacy. *Neurology* (abstract), 36 (supp):100–101, 1986.

Saper JR. Changing perspectives in headache treatment. *Clin J Pain*, 2:19–29, 1986.

Saper JR. Daily chronic headache, tension headache, migraine, and combined headache: The transformation concept. (In) *Drug-Induced Headache*. HC Diener and M Wilkinson (Eds), Berlin, Springer-Verlag, 1988.

Saper JR. Ergotamine dependency: A review. *Headache*, 27:435–438, 1987.

Chapter 10

Caviness VS Jr., O'Brien P. Cluster headache response to chlorpromazine. *Headache*, 20:128–131, 1980.

Diamond S, Dalessio DG. *The Practicing Physician's Approach to Headache*. Fifth edition. Baltimore, Williams & Wilkins, 1992.

Ekbom K, Lindgren L, Nilsson BY, et al. Retro-gasserian glycerol injection in the treatment of chronic cluster headache. *Cephalalgia*, 7:21–27, 1987.

Fogan L. Treatment of cluster headache. A double-blind comparison of oxygen vs. air inhalation. *Arch Neurol*, 42:362–363, 1985.

Fusco BM, Geppetti P, Fancicullaci M, et al. Local application of capsaicin for treatment of cluster headache and idiopathic trigeminal neuralgia. *Cephalalgia*, 11 (supp 2):234–245, 1991.

Gabe IJ, Spierings CLH. Prophylactic treatment of cluster headache with verapamil. *Headache*, 29:167–168, 1989.

Herring R, Kuritzky A. Sodium valproate in the treatment of cluster headache: An open label trial. *Cephalalgia*, 9:195–198, 1989.

Jammes JJ. The treatment of cluster headache with prednisone. *Diseased Nervous System*, 36:375–376, 1975.

Jotkowitz S. Chronic paroxysmal hemicrania and cluster. *Ann Neurol*, 4:389, 1978.

Kudrow L, Kudrow DB. Association of systemic oxyhemoglobin desaturation and onset of cluster headache attacks. *Headache*, 30:474–480, 1990.

Kudrow L. *Cluster Headache Mechanisms and Management*. London, Oxford University Press, 1980.

Kudrow L. Response of cluster headache attack to oxygen inhalation. *Headache*, 21:1–4, 1981.

Mathew NT, Hurt W. Percutaneous radiofrequency trigeminal gangliorhyzolysis in intractable cluster headache. *Headache*, 28:328–331, 1988.

Mathew NT, Ruevini U. Cluster-like headache following head trauma. *Headache*, (abstract), 28:307, 1988.

Mathew NT. Advances in cluster headache. (In) *Neurologic Clinics*, NT Mathew (Ed). Pgs 867–890, November, 1990.

Mathew NT. Cluster headache. *Neurology*, 42 (supp 2):22–31, 1992.

Mathew NT. Cluster headache. *Intractable Headache: Inpatient and Outpatient Treatment Strategies*. SD Silberstein (Ed), Neurology 42 (supp 2):22–31, 1992.

Maxwell RE. Surgical control of chronic migrainous neuralgia by trigeminal gangliorhyzolysis. *J Neurol Surg*, 57:459–466, 1982.

Moskowitz MA. Cluster headache: Evidence for a pathophysiological focus in the superior pericarotid cavernous sinus plexus. *Headache*, 28:584–586, 1988.

Onofrio BM, Campbell JK. Surgical treatment of chronic cluster headache. Mayo Clinic Proceedings, 61:537–544, 1986.

Sjaastad O, Apfelbaum R, Caskey W, et al. Chronic paroxysmal hemicrania (CPH): The clinical manifestation. A review. *Ups J Med Sci* (suppl), 31:27–33, 1980.

Sjaastad O, Fredriksen TA, Pfraffenrath V. The cervicogenic headache: Diagnostic criteria. *Headache*, 30:725–726, 1990.

Sjaastad O. Chronic paroxysmal hemicrania. (In) *Handbook of Clinical Neurology*, Vol. 48. FC Rose (Ed). Amsterdam, Elsevier Science Publishing, pgs 257–266, 1986.

Sjaastad O. Cluster headache. (In) *Handbook of Clinical Neurology*, Vol. 48. FC Rose (Ed). Amsterdam, Elsevier Science Publishing, pgs 217–246, 1986.

Solomon S, Apfelbaum RI, Guglielmo KM. The cluster-tic syndrome and its surgical treatment. *Cephalalgia*, 5:83–89, 1985.

Watson CPN, Morley TP, Richardson JC, et al. The surgical treatment of chronic cluster headache. *Headache*, 23:289–895, 1985.

Chapter 11

Arner S, Lindplom U, Meyerson BA, et al. Prolonged relief of neuralgia after regional anesthetic blocks: A call for further experimental and systematic clinical studies. *Pain*, 43:287–297, 1990.

Bindoff LA, Heseltine D. Unilateral face pain in patients with lung cancer. Referred pain via the vagus. *Lancet*, 1:812–815, 1988.

Bogduk N. Greater occipital neuralgia. (In) DM Long (ed). *Current Therapy in Neurological Surgery*, Toronto, B.C. Decker, pgs 175–180, 1985.

Bogduk N. Local anesthetic blocks of the second cervical ganglion: A technique with application in occipital headache. *Cephalalgia*, 1:41–50, 1981.

Bogduk N, Marsland A. On the concept of third occipital headache. *J Neurol Neurosurg Psychiatry*, 49:775–780, 1986.

Bovim G, Berg R, Dale LG. Cervicogenic headache: Anesthetic blockades of cervical nerves. (C2-C5) and facet joint (C2/C3). *Pain*, 49:315–20, 1992a.

Bovim G, Fredriksen TA, Stolt-Nielsen A, Sjaastad O. Neurolysis of the greater occipital nerve in cervicogenic headache. A follow-up study. *Headache*, 32:175–9, 1992b.

Bruyn GW. Glossopharyngeal neuralgia. (In) *Handbook of Clinical Neurology*, Vol. 48. FC Rose (Ed). Amsterdam, Elsevier Science Publishers, pgs 459–473, 1986.

Burchiel KJ, Clark EH, Haglund M, et al. Long-term efficacy of microvascular decompression of trigeminal neuralgia. *J Neurosurg*, 69:35–38, 1988.

Chawla JC, Falconer MA. Glossopharyngeal and vagal neuralgia. *Brit Med J*, 3:529–531, 1967.

Cooper BC, Rabuzzi DD. Myofascial pain dysfunction syndrome: A clinical study of asymptomatic subjects. *Laryngoscope*, 94:68–75, 1984.

Court JE, Case CS. Treatment of tic douloureux with anticonvulsant (clonazapam). *J Neurol Neurosurg Psychiatry*, 39:297–299, 1976.

Denny-Brown D, Adams RD, Fitzgerald PJ. Pathologic features of herpes zoster: A note on "geniculate herpes." *Arch Neurol Psychiatry*, 51:216–231, 1944.

Druce HM, Slavin RG. Sinusitis: Critical need for further study. *J Allergy Clin Immunol*, 88:675–677, 1991.

Dwyer A, Aprill C, Bogduk N. Cervical zygapophyseal joint pain patterns I. A study in normal volunteers. *Spine*, 15:453–457, 1990.

Ekbom KA, Westerburg CE. Carbamazepine in glossopharyngeal neuralgia. *Arch Neurol*, 14:595–596, 1966.

Fromm GH, Terrence CF, Chattha AS. Baclofen in the treatment of trigeminal neuralgia: Double-blind study and long-term follow-up. *Ann Neurol*, 15:240–244, 1984.

Goadsby PJ, Zagami AS, Lambert GA. Neuroprocessing of craniovascular pain: A synthesis of the central structures involved in migraine. *Headache*, 31:365–371, 1991.

Graff-Radford SB. Oral mandibular disorders and headache: A critical appraisal. (In) *Neurologic Clinics*, NT Mathew (Ed). Pgs 929–943, November, 1990.

Graff-Radford SB, Reeves JL, Jagger B. Management of chronic head and neck pain: Effectiveness of altering factors perpetuating myofascial pain. *Headache*, 27:186–190, 1987.

Janetta PJ. Microsurgical management of trigeminal neuralgia. *Arch Neurol*, 42:800, 1985.

Kerr FWL. Central relationships of trigeminal and cervical primary afferents in the spinal cord and medulla. *Brain Res*, 43:561–572, 1972.

Lance JW, Anthony M. Neck-tongue syndrome on sudden turning of the head. *J Neurol Neurosurg Psychiatry*, 43:97–101, 1980.

Lechin F, Vanderdigs B, Lechin ME, et al. Pimozide therapy for trigeminal neuralgia. *Arch Neurol*, 9:960–964, 1989.

Leijon G, Boivia J, Johansson I. Central post-stroke pain. Neurological symptoms and pain characteristics. *Pain*, 36:13–25, 1989.

Margolis MT, Stein RL, Newton DH. Extracranial aneurysms of the internal carotid artery. *Neuroradiology*, 4:78–89, 1972.

Mehigan JT, Olcott C. Carotidynia associated with carotid arterial disease and stroke. *Am J Surg*, 142:210–211, 1981.

McNamara RM, O'Brien MC, David-Heiser S. Post-traumatic neck pain: A prospective and follow-up study. *Ann Emerg Med*, 17:906–911, 1988.

Portenoy RK, Duma C, Foley KM. Acute herpetic and post-herpetic neuralgia: Clinical review and current management. *Ann Neurol*, 20:651–664, 1986.

Raskin NH, Prusiner S. Carotidynia. *Neurology*, 27:43–46, 1977.

Raskin NH, Schwartz RK. Icepick-like pain. *Neurology*, 30:203–205, 1980.

Ratner EJ, Langer B, Evins ML. Alveolar cavitational osteoporosis. *J Periodont*, 57:593–603, 1986.

Ratner EJ, Person P, Kleinman DJ, et al. Jawbone cavities in trigeminal and atypical facial neuralgias. *Oral Surg*, 48:3–20, 1979.

Rittenhouse EA, Radke HM, Sumner DS. Carotid artery aneurysm. *Arch Surg*, 105:786–789, 1972.

Sessle BJ, Hu JW, Amano N, Zhong G. Convergence of cutaneous, tooth pulp, visceral, neck, and muscle afferents onto nociceptive and non-nociceptive neurons in trigeminal subnucleus caudalis (medullary dorsal horn) and its implications for referred pain. *Pain*, 27:219–235, 1986.

Sicuteri F, Nicolodi M, Fusco BM, Orlando S. Idiopathic headache as a possible risk factor for phantom tooth pain. *Headache*, 31:577–581, 1981.

Solomon S, Lipton RB. Facial pain. (In) *Neurologic Clinics*, NT Mathew (Ed). Pgs 913–928, November, 1990.

Sweet WH. The treatment of trigeminal neuralgia. *New Engl J Med*, 316:692–693, 1987.

Swerdlow M. Anticonvulsant drugs and chronic pain. *Clin Neuropharmacol*, 7:51–82, 1984.

Wallin BJ, Westerberg CE, Sundlof G. Syncope induced by glossopharyngeal neuralgia: Sympathetic outflow to muscle. *Neurology*, 34:522–524, 1984.

Waltz TA, Dalessio DJ, Copeland B, et al. Percutaneous injection of glycerol for the treatment of trigeminal neuralgia. *Clin J Pain*, 5:195–198, 1989.

Watson CPN, Evans RJ, Reed K, et al. Amitriptyline vs. placebo in postherpetic neuralgic. *Neurology*, 32:671–673, 1982.

Watson CPN, Evans RJ. Treatment of post-herpetic neuralgia. *Clin Neuropharmacol*, 9:533–541, 1986B.

Watson CPN, Evans RJ. Post-herpetic neuralgia: A review. *Arch Neurol*, 43:836–840, 1986A.

Yarri Y, Selzer ME, Pincus JH. Phenytoin: Mechanisms of anticonvulsant action. *Ann Neurol*, 20:171–184, 1986.

Chapter 12

Carlsson GS, Svardsudd K, Wellin L. Long-term effects of head injury sustained during life in three male populations. *J Neurosurg*, 67:197–205, 1987.

Dila C, Bouchard L, Myer E, Yamamoto L, Feindel W. Microvascular response to minimal brain trauma. (In) *Head Injuries*, R McLaurin (Ed). Grune & Stratton, New York, 1976.

Dillon H, Leopold RL. Children and the post-concussion syndrome. *JAMA*, 175:86–92, 1961.

Feinsod M, Hoyt WF, Wilson WG, Spire JP. Visual evoked response: Use in neurological evaluation of post-traumatic subjective visual complaints. *Arch Ophthalmol*, 94:237–240, 1976.

Fisher CM. Whiplash amnesia. *Neurology*, 32:667–668, 1982.

Gennareli TA. Cerebral concussion and diffuse brain injuries. (In) *Head Injury*, PR Cooper (Ed). Baltimore, Williams & Wilkins, pgs 83–97, 1982.

Gronwall D, Wrightson P. Delayed recovery of intellectual function after minor head injury. *Lancet*, 2:605–609, 1984.

Haas DC, Pineda GS, Lourie H. Juvenile head trauma syndromes and their relationship to migraine. *Arch Neurol*, 32:727–730, 1975.

Jacome DE. Basilar artery migraine after uncomplicated whiplash injuries. *Headache*, 26:515–516, 1986.

Jakobsen J, Daadsgaard SE, Thomsen S, et al. Prediction of post-concussional sequelae by reaction time test. *Acta Neurol Scandinavia*, 75:341–345, 1987.

Keith WS. Whiplash injury of the second cervical ganglion and nerve. *Can J Neurolog Sci*, 13:133–137, 1986.

Kelly R. The post-traumatic syndrome. *Proc Royal Soc Med*, 24:242–244, 1981.

Kerr FWL. A mechanism to account for frontal headache in a case of posterior fossa tumors. *J Neurosurg*, 18:605–609, 1961.

Khurana RK, Nirankari VW. Bilateral sympathetic dysfunction in posttraumatic headache. *Headache*, 26:183–188, 1986.

Klonoff PS, Snow WE, Costa LD. Quality of life in patients 2–4 years after closed head injury. *Neurosurgery*, 19:735–743, 1986.

Leininger BE. Neuropsychological deficits in symptomatic minor head injury patients after concussion and mild concussion. *J Neurol Neurosurg Psychiatry*, 53:293–296, 1990.

MacFlynn G, Montgomery EA, Fenton GW, Rutherford DW. Measurement of reaction time following minor head injury. *J Neurol Neurosurg Psychiatry*, 47:1326–1331, 1984.

Matthews WB. Footballer's migraine, *Brit Med J*, 2:326–327, 1972.

McKinley WW, Brooks DN, Bond MR. Post-concussional symptoms, financial compensation, and outcome of severe blunt head injury. *J Neurol Neurosurg Psychiatry*, 46:1084–1091, 1983.

Merskey H, Woodforde JM. Psychiatric sequelae of minor head injury. *Brain*, 95:521–528, 1972.

Noseworthy JH, Miller J, Murray TJ, Regan D. Auditory brainstem responses in post-concussion syndrome. *Arch Neurol*, 389:275–278, 1981.

Ommaya AK, Faas F, Yarnell P. Whiplash injury and brain damage: An experimental study. *JAMA*, 204:275–289, 1968.

Oppenheimer DR. Microscopic lesions in the brain following head injury. *J Neurol Neurosurg Psychiatry*, 31:299–306, 1968.

Povlishok JT, Becker DP, Cheng CLY, et al. Axonal changes in minor head injury. *J Neuropathol, Experimental Neurol*, 42:225–242, 1983.

Raskin NH. *Headache*. Churchill-Livingstone, New York, 1988.

Rimel RW, Giordani B, Barth JT, et al. Disability caused by minor head injury. *Neurosurgery*, 9:221–228, 1981.

Rizzo PA, Pierelli F, Pozzessere G, et al. Subjective post-traumatic syndrome: A comparison of visual and brainstem auditory evoked responses. *Neuropsychobiology*, 9:78–82, 1983.

Rowe JM, Carlson C. Brainstem auditory evoked potential in post-concussion dizziness. *Arch Neurol*, 37:679–683, 1980.

Sackallares JC, Giordani B, Berent S, et al. Patients with pseudoseizures: intellectual and cognitive performance. *Neurology*, 35:116–119, 1985.

Smith RG, Cherry JE. Traumatic Eagle's syndrome: Report of a case and review of the literature. *J Oral Maxillofacial Surg*, 46:606–609, 1988.

Starkstein SE, Mayberg HS, Bertwier ML, et al. Mania after brain injury: Neuroradiological and metabolic findings. *Ann Neurol*, 27:652–659, 1990.

Stuss DT, Ely P, Hugenholtz H, Richard MT, et al. Subtle neuropsychological deficits in patients with good recovery after closed head injury. *Neurosurgery*, 17:41–47, 1985.

Symonds CP. Mental disorder following head injury. *Proc Royal Soc Med*, 30:1081, 1937.

Tarsh MJ, Royston C. A follow-up study of accident neurosis. *Brit J Psychiatry*, 146:18–25, 1985.

Toglia JU, Rosenberg PE, Ronis ML. Post-traumatic dizziness. *Arch Otolaryngol*, 92:485–492, 1970.

Torres F, Shapiro SK. Electroencephalograms and whiplash injury. *Arch Neurol*, 5:40–47, 1961.

Trimbell MR. *Post-traumatic Neurosis: From Railway Spine to the Whiplash.* New York, John Wiley and Sons, 1981.

Vijayan N, Dreyfus PM. Post-traumatic dysautonomic cephalgia. *Arch Neurol*, 32:649–652, 1975.

Wei EP, Dietrich WD, Polvichek JT, et al. Functional, morphological, and metabolic abnormalities of the cerebral microcirculation after concussive brain injury in cats. *Circ Res*, 46:37–47, 1980.

West M, LaBella FS, Havlicek V, et al. Cerebral concussion in rats rapidly induces hypothalamic-specific effects on opiate and cholinergic receptors. *Brain Res*, 25:271–277, 1981.

Winston KR. Whiplash and its relationship to migraine. *Headache*, 27:452–457, 1987.

Chapter 13

Bank H. Idiopathic carotiditis. *Lancet*, 1:726, 1978.

Cox LK, Bertorini T, Lassiter RE. Headaches due to spontaneous internal carotid artery dissection: Magnetic resonance imaging evaluation follow-up. *Headache*, 31:12–16, 1991.

Fisher CM. The headache and pain of spontaneous carotid dissection. *Headache*, 22:660–665, 1982.

Hart RG, Easton JD. Dissections of cervical and cerebral arteries. *Neurolog Clin*, 1:155–182, 1983.

Mehigan JT, Olcott C. Carotidynia associated with carotid arterial disease and stroke. *Am J Surg*, 142:210–211, 1981.

Mokri B, Sundt TM, Houser OW, et al. Spontaneous dissection of the cervical internal artery. *Ann Neurol*, 19:126–138, 1986.

Orfei R, Meienberg O. Carotidynia: Report of eight cases and prospective evaluation of therapy. *J Neurol*, 230:65–72, 1983.

Raskin NH, Prusiner S. Carotidynia. *Neurology*, 27:43–46, 1977.

Rittenhouse EA, Radke HM, Sumner DS. Carotid artery aneurysm. *Arch Surg*, 105:786–789, 1972.

Rothrock JF, Lim V, Press G, Gosink B. Serial magnetic resonance and carotid duplex examinations in the management of carotid dissection. *Neurology*, 38:686–692, 1989.

Chapter 14

Akpunonu BE, Ahrens J. Sexual headaches: Case report. Review and treatment with calcium blocker. *Headache*, 31:141–145, 1991.

Bordini C, Gantonaci F, Stovner J, et al. Hemicrania continua: A clinical review. *Headache*, 31:20–26, 1991.

Braun A, Klawans HL. Headaches associated with exercise and sexual activity. (In) *Handbook of Clinical Neurology*, Vol. 48. FC Rose (Ed). Amsterdam, Elsevier Science Publishers, pgs 373–382, 1986.

Ekbom K. Cough headache. (In) *Handbook of Clinical Neurology*, Vol. 48. FC Rose (Ed). Amsterdam, Elsevier Science Publishers, pgs 367–371, 1986.

Hannerz J, Ericson K, Bergstrand G. Chronic paroxysmal hemicrania: Orbital phlebography and steroid treatment. *Cephalalgia*, 7:189–192, 1987.

Johns DR. Benign sexual headache within a family. *Arch Neurol*, 43:1158–1160, 1986.

Kuritzky A. Indomethacin-resistant hemicrania continua. *Cephalalgia*, 12:57–59, 1992.

Paulson GW, Klawans HL. Benign orgasmic cephalgia. *Headache*, 13:181–187, 1974.

Porter M, Jankovic J. Benign coital cephalgia: Differential diagnosis and treatment. *Arch Neurol*, 38:710–712, 1981.

Raskin NH. *Headache*. Churchill-Livingstone, New York, 1988.

Rooke ED. Benign exertional headache. *Med Clin North Amer*, 52:801–808, 1968.

Russel D. Chronic paroxysmal hemicrania: Severity, duration, and time of occurrence of attacks. *Cephalalgia*, 4:53–56, 1984.

Selwyn DL. A study of coital-related headaches in 32 patients. *Cephalalgia*, 5 (supp 3):300–301, 1985.

Sjaastad O. Chronic paroxysmal hemicrania. (In) *Handbook of Clinical Neurology*, Vol. 48. FC Rose (Ed). Amsterdam, Elsevier Science Publishers, pgs 257–266, 1986.

Sjaastad O, Dale I. Evidence for a new (?) treatable headache entity. *Headache*, 14:105–108, 1974.

Sjaastad O, Spierings ELH. "Hemicrania continua:" Another headache absolutely responsive to indomethacin. *Cephalalgia*, 4:65–70, 1984.

Chapter 15

Khurana RK. Headache spectrum and Arnold-Chiari malformation. *Headache*, 31:151–155, 1991.

Marcelis J, Silberstein SD. Idiopathic intracranial hypertension without papilledema. *Arch Neurol*, 48:392–396, 1991.

Marcelis J, Silberstein SD. Spontaneous low cerebral spinal fluid pressure headache. *Headache*, 30:192–196, 1190.

Matthew RJ, Wilson WH. Caffeine-induced changes in cerebral circulation. *Stroke*, 16:814–817, 1985.

Sechzer PG, Abel L. Post-spinal anesthesia headache treated with caffeine: Evaluation with demand method. Part I. *Curr Ther Res*, 24:307–312, 1978.

Seebacher J, Ribeiro V, LeGuillou JL, et al. Epidural blood patch in the treatment of post-dural puncture headache: A double-blind study. *Headache*, 29:630–632, 1989.

Silberstein SD, Marcelis J. Headache associated with changes in intracranial pressure. *Headache*, 32:84–94, 1992.

Chapter 16

Aisenberg RM, Rottenberg DA. The pathogenesis of pseudotumor cerebri. *J Neurol Sci*, 48:51–60, 1980.

Black PM, Conner ES. Chronic increased intracranial pressure. (In) *Disease of the Nervous System*. AK Asbury, GM McKhann, WI McDonald (Eds). Philadelphia, W.B. Saunders, pgs 1053–1063, 1986.

Bortoluzzi M, DiLauro L, Marini G. Benign intracranial hypertension with spinal and radicular pain. *J Neurosurg* 57:833–836, 1982.

Corbett JJ, Jacobson DM, Thompson HS, Hart MN, et al. Results of optic nerve sheath fenestration for pseudotumor cerebri. *Arch Neurol*, 106:1391–1397, 1988.

Hart RG, Carter JE. Pseudotumor cerebri and facial pain. *Arch Neurol*, 39:440–441, 1982.

Raskin NH. *Headache*. Churchill-Livingstone, New York, 1988.

Round R, Keene J. The minor symptoms of increased intracranial pressure: 101 patients with benign intracranial hypertension. *Neurology*, 38:1461–1464, 1988.

Sorensen PS, Krogsaa B, Jerris G. Clinical course and prognosis of pseudotumor cerebri: A prospective study of 24 patients. *Acta Neurolog Scand*, 77:164–172, 1988.

Chapter 17

Aprill C, Dwyer A, Bogduk N. Cervical zygapophyseal joint pain patterns II: A clinical evaluation. *Spine*, 15:458–461, 1990.

Arner S, Lindbolm U, Meyerson BA, et al. Prolonged relief of neuralgia after regional anesthetic blocks: A call for further experimental and systemic clinical studies. *Pain*, 43:287–297, 1990.

Bogduk N. Local anesthetic blocks of the second cervical ganglion: Technique with application in occipital headache. *Cephalalgia*, 1:41–50, 1981.

Bogduk N. The clinical anatomy of the cervical dorsal rami. *Spine*, 7:319–330, 1982.

Bovim G, Berg R, Dale LG. Cervicogenic headache: Anesthetic blockades of cervical nerves (C2-C5) and facet joint (C2/C3). *Pain*, 49:315–320, 1992a.

Bovim G, Fredriksen TA, Stolt-Nielsen A, Sjaastad O. Neurolysis of the greater occipital nerve in cervicogenic headache. A follow-up study. *Headache*, 32:175–179, 1992b.

Busch E, Wilson PR. Atlanto-occipital and atlanto-axial injections in the treatment of headache and neck pain. *Reg Anaesth*, 14 (supp 2):45, 1989.

Dwyer A, Aprill C, Bogduk N. Cervical zygapophyseal joint patterns I: A study in normal volunteers. *Spine*, 15:453–457, 1990.

Ehni G, Benner B. Occipital neuralgia in C1-C2 arthrosis syndrome. *J Neurosurg*, 61:961–965, 1984.

Gawel MJ, Rothbart PJ. Occipital nerve block in the management of headache and cervical pain. *Cephalalgia*, 12:9–13, 1992.

Gore DR, Sepic FB, Gardner GM, Murray MP. Neck pain: A long-term follow-up of 205 patients. *Spine*, 12:1–5, 1987.

Graff-Radford SB, Reeves JL, Jaeger B. Management of chronic head and neck pain: Effectiveness of altering factors perpetuating myofascial pain. *Headache*, 27:186–190, 1987.

Keith WS. "Whiplash" injury of the second cervical ganglion and nerve. *Can J Neurolog Sci*, 13:133–137, 1986.

Kerr FWL. A mechanism to account for frontal headache in cases of posterior fossa tumors. *J Neurosurg*, 18:605–609, 1961.

Kerr FWL. Central relationships of trigeminal and cervical primary aferrents in the cord and medulla. *Brain Res*, 43:561–572, 1972.

Lamer TJ. Ear pain due to cervical spine arthritis: Treatment with cervical facet injection. *Headache*, 31:682–683, 1991.

LaRocca H. Cervical sprain syndrome: Diagnosis, treatment, and long-term outcome. (In) *The Adult Spine: Principles and Practices*. JW Frymoyer (Ed). New York, Raven Press, pg 1051, 1991.

McNamera RM, O'Brien MC, Davidheizer S. Post-traumatic neck pain: A prospective and follow-up study. *Ann Emerg Med*, 17:906–911, 1988.

Olesen J. Clinical and pathophysiological observations in migraine and tension-type headache explained by integration of vascular, supraspinal, and myofascial input. *Pain*, 46:125–132, 1991.

Travell JG, Dimons DJ. Posterior cervical muscles: Semispinalis capitis, semispinalis cervices, and multifidi: "Pain in the neck." (In) *Myofascial Pain and Dysfunction: The Trigger Point Manual* JG Travell, Simons DG (Eds). Baltimore, Williams & Wilkins, pg 305, 1983.

Winston KR. Whiplash and its relationship to migraine. *Headache*, 27:452–467, 1987.

Index